ON THE
OTHER
SIDE

ON THE OTHER SIDE

A BROWN GIRL'S JOURNEY
TO FIND HOPE THROUGH DEPRESSION

✖ ✖ ✖ ✖ ✖

SANDI TREVINO RAE

✖ ✖ ✖ ✖ ✖

ACKNOWLEDGMENTS

Writing this book was so much harder than I had imagined, but also so much more rewarding than expected. It could not have been possible without the strong role model and love of my mother, Grace. She showed me how to be true to my Mexican heritage and to be proud of being a woman in this tough world of ours. I also need to thank my incredible children, Joshua, Nicole, and Anne, who taught me the true meaning of loving unconditionally and without judgment. You taught your mom how precious life can be and I am blessed by each of you daily. You are truly my greatest gifts.

I am eternally grateful to "the Minnesota Babes", my Tonna book club women, and to my book launch leader/web designer/dear friend, Bethany-I could not have completed this journey without any of you. Your prayers, love, and support got my through the times of doubt and delight. Thank you to Jeremy and the team at Book Boss for helping me bring my manuscript to life.

To my Dan, what can I say? You my sweet guy have been my biggest cheerleader, my confidant, and the one to say "you can't give up now; you have a message to tell." Through all the late nights scanning re-writes and early morning coffees listening to me reading new excerpts, you have encouraged me and been my safe place to land, thank you my love.

And lastly, to all the Occupational Therapists and other health professionals that reach out to care for those of us dealing with mental illness, you show kindness, patience, and God's love without fail. You are my heroes and you save lives like mine every day. Thank you.

TABLE OF CONTENTS

Summary

PROLOGUE

THE PRECURSOR TO TONIGHT'S PROCEEDINGS

"What mental health needs is more sunlight, more candor, and more unashamed conversation."

—Glenn Close

Thank you, dear reader, for being here. It means the world to me. It may also mean you have been through some pretty tough times and have had your share of struggles on your journey too.

This is a book written for any person who suffers from or may know someone who may suffer from mental illness. This is not your typical self-help book. It is full of good humor, positivity, and real talk. This book will guide you through the world of mental health, with a peppering of my own experiences working in mental health institutions and then being admitted as a patient into one. It's a unique, colorful, heartbreaking story at times, but one which ends with hope for the future. Focusing on the mental health battle from a professional perspective, but I also share my own personal story with you in the hope that it can support you through tough times, help you to know that you're not alone, and open dialogue about mental health and self-care.

Mental health should not be taboo; it should be as easy to talk about as a headache. Mental illness is an *illness*! Let me repeat that for the people in the back... Mental illness is an *illness*. It is valid. It is real. If you're lucky enough to have never struggled with your own mental health, then I hope you continue to stick with this book. It will provide you with tools and perspective for good days and not so good days. My hope is that you too may gain hope from listening to my story. It is very hard to explain what a mental illness feels like to somebody else, but I'm going to try. This is my story, my experience. Everyone's journey is different. My journey although personal and vulnerable at times, sharing this with you is a cathartic process. I can cope with being honest and a little red-faced by the end of it if it means that my book sparks a conversation surrounding mental health.

You can expect a smattering of my own poetry throughout the book. Poetry is a guilty little pleasure that helps me process my feelings and experiences. And I have had my share. Before we dive headfirst into the vast ocean of mental health, let me leave you with a poem about mental health and how it feels to me to bear the weight of a hidden injury. Because that's what mental health issues can feel like—hidden injuries, ones that lie just below the surface, unseen but oh so painful.

The Hidden Injury

———————

Why can't I turn my head when I see a car crash?
I seem to hope that I see blood and guts. Is that wrong?
I have suffered from depression for thirty-four years, but it
does not show on the outside. I could be in a
very bad place, a crash. But it does not show. No blood, no guts, and no second looks,
and most distressing, no compassion.

No one says, "Oh, I feel so bad, she has mental illness."
Instead, people stay away and look away. Don't
they know it's not contagious?

———————

In each chapter throughout this book, and sprinkled around the pages like glitter, I'll include quotes from various people that speak to me personally. You'll notice that not all of the words of wisdom I include are positive, because we can't all be positive all of the time. Toxic positivity is not what we need in our lives. What we need are real talks, real stories, real recoveries. That's what you'll get from me in this book. I won't sugarcoat things and make everything seem sweet and easy. You'll soon find out that I'm not one to censor my experiences nor my feelings about things. One thing I will guarantee is that this book won't be heavy, however. You won't feel drained the way some self-help books make you feel. I hope that you'll feel like you've nestled into a comfy chair and shared a cup of warm coffee with a friend—a friend who's a little blunt, a little broken, but real. None of us are perfect, and I'm more than happy to share the chips in my china with you. You'll also have the chance to jot down some of your own thoughts and feelings too. This may help you to feel more engaged in your own journey.

Let me share a little about me before we grab shovels and truly dig into who I am in the next chapter…

I really don't like people. Is that wrong of me to say? Let me stat over. I don't like mean people. Okay, now may get cozy and curl up and read my touching story. I have had brown skin my whole life. I have felt fat or too curvy for many years of my life. I have had mental illness most of my life. I have been divorced and lonely too. And mean people have been there kicking me when I was down and letting me know I was not okay through-out all of those struggles. Believe me, this is not a "feel sorry for me, I'm a victim" book. I am simply saying, "There is absolutely no room for mean folks on this train."

Being okay and feeling worthy has been my goal for as long as I can remember. My parents divorced when I was four years old. I remember not understanding as I would look up at my mother's dark porcelain face with tears flowing down her cheeks. "What happened? Why are you sad, momma?" Little did I know that my whole world was about to change. My papa was never coming home again.

I grew up in a small town in southern Minnesota, better known as blond-hair, blue-eyed country. My mother moved from Texas to Minnesota to be near my grandparents after she divorced my father. My mom talks about how alone she felt but how strong she needed to be now for her little girls. She had to make a living and make our world whole again. My mother is one of the strongest women I have ever known. As I grew up, I watched as she built her dream of running a restaurant of her own, only to have to pick up the pieces of a destroyed dream when her restaurant was vandalized, as she was called terrible, filthy names because of the color of her skin, and as she lived as a single mom in a world of two-parent families. She prevailed; she kept her head high. She had a dream to convert lutefisk- and lefsa-eating Minnesotans to burrito-loving consumers. It really is okay, Lutherans, to eat tacos after church on Sunday. God will still love you. My momma had a job to do and that was to make a world for her two little girls. And that world was going to happen in Minnesota. But there will be more about this in the next chapter. For now, what you need to know is that I had a strong mother as a role model, yet I was no match against the power of mental illness. It's always been there in the background, darkness creeping and stalking me.

I credit my personal experiences with mental health as the reason I decided to work in that field. I've worked on so many different psychiatric units and with so many different patients. I love the jobs I've had. One example is my experience when I was working in mental health in a women's prison. As a five-foot, four-inch little Mexican girl, I was naïve and a wide-eyed doe compared to those street-wise inmates, but I treated them all with respect, and that made all the difference. No matter where I work, it feels like I'm doing something worthwhile, having carried baggage of my own. I have an idea what these inmates and what my patients may be going through, and this helps me to help them. I may not have walked in their shoes or on their particular paths, but I have slid my feet into many a sandal and traveled down similar roads and walkways. Going from being the occupational therapist (OT) leading group therapy sessions in secure units to being admitted to one is a steep learning curve.

✖ ✖ ✖ ✖ ✖

THERE IS STILL A STIGMA AROUND MENTAL HEALTH

I t would be silly for us to pretend otherwise. After all, if there was no stigma then I wouldn't be here writing this book, coffee in hand and memories flooding my brain.

Glenn Close, the incredible actor who frightened us all with "the bunny incident" absolutely hit the nail on the head with these words. They encapsulate the very essence of this book: "What mental health needs is more sunlight, more candor, more unashamed conversation about illnesses that affect not only individuals, but their families as well."

If you thought the stigma was bad simply around mental health, it is magnified tenfold as soon as the person suffering is a parent. As you may already be aware, one large priority within mental health as a whole, and a huge passion personally, is around parents with mental health issues. This area hits very close to home; it actually was my home, my hiding place, for years. I still find that this is swept under the rug, but that is unfair! With such large numbers of children growing up with parents who have mental health issues, it makes me want to pull my hair out that more people aren't talking about this and reaching out for help!

There is so much that can be done to minimize the impact a parent's mental illness has on a child, and simply acknowledging that this is real and absolutely normal allows for us as a society to move to protect the parents and children. Being a parent with a mental illness does not make you a bad parent. It does not make you any worse than any other parent out there. I can personally attest to this! I think I was, and still am, a good mother not only in spite of my mental illness but possibly because of it too. I am a firm believer that people who have suffered from mental illness have a wealth of knowledge and experience to share because of their experience. They have insight that others may never be privy to know. Every cloud has a silver lining, right? Being a mother with a mental illness with trials and overcoming those trials helped me in teaching my children about trials and perseverance when raising my own children; that silver lining was bedazzled and shiny. With a third of children growing up with a parent with a mental illness, I can't wrap my head around how this is still a taboo subject.[1] While there are a couple of areas in this book that focus on parenting, most of the book is quite generic and can apply to everyone.

It is worth pointing out here that everyone may experience characteristics of mental illness occasionally, but if you find that

1 "Parental mental ill-health," Safeguarding Network, accessed February 28, 2021, https://safeguarding. network/safeguarding-resources/parental-issues/parental-mental-ill-health/.

you're experiencing them fairly regularly, or a few of them at once, further evaluation is likely to be helpful for you. Disclaimer alert! If you have suicidal thoughts or ideations, this is the time to seek medical attention. I know how hard it can be to admit it, and to put yourself out there for treatment, but you need to do it. I'll share my story with you momentarily, and how my experience with mental illness and suicidal thoughts fit into my narrative, but I just need to put out there into the world that suicidal thoughts are not something you shrug off. Maybe somebody reading this just needed to be reminded, and that's okay. Just think of me as the lady who's been there, done that, and got the T-shirt. You'll be able to identify a few red flags throughout my story; believe me, they are everywhere. At times in my life, I lived in a sea of solid ruby red flags surrounding me. I hope that this will allow you to identify if you have some red flags in your own life or maybe if a loved one does. Identifying and acknowledging difficulties is half of the battle.

✖ ✖ ✖ ✖ ✖

WHAT SHOULD YOU EXPECT FROM THE REST OF THE BOOK?

Well, the next chapter is all about me! The good, the bad, and the ugly. No holds barred. The truth, the whole truth, and nothing but the truth. I'm past the point in my life where I feel the need to hide my struggles and my achievements (because I do have some of those too). So, expect a story about a little brown girl living in Minnesota trying her best to fit in. You'll follow my story through the ups and downs, with some poetry and quotes thrown in for good measure. By sharing my story I hope to encourage other people to share their own.

"It's so common, it could be anyone. The trouble is, nobody wants to talk about it. And that makes everything worse."

—Ruby Wax

Then we get into the good stuff. The helpful, practical stuff, with my own little Sandi-isms. Being a woman working on psychiatric units, and then being admitted to one, gives me a certain insight. I like to think it gives me an edge. What once brought me down is now one of my strongest attributes. This experience helps me to help you, and that's what I want to do. I want to help make the world a little bit brighter. My self-help might not be the typical self-help you see, but I think that's what makes it useful! After years of working as an occupational therapist and personally traveling down dark roads of depression, I learned a few things that have brought glimpses of hope and joy to myself and to others.

Poems from my darkest periods teach me that things get better. What was once broken can be fixed.

Smaller, smaller, then gone
——————

I try to be perfect, try to be all they want.
I would choose all the right answers and get an A plus.
I try to be thinnest, the girl with the least,
The number on the scale is the trophy I want most.
I try to be perfect, try to be all they want.
I would score all the goals, make the team and coach proud.
I try to be smaller, try to shrink if I can,
I would choose invisible, just gone if I could.
I try to be smaller, the smallest is key,
I would choose a small casket, make me happiest for good.

——————

What do you hope to gain from this book? You could write personal reflection or just a few thoughts.

_____

_____

_____

_____

_____

_____

_____

_____

_____

_____

_____

_____

_____

_____

_____

_____

_____

_____

_____

_____

MY STORY: ON THE OTHER SIDE

HOW I ENDED UP IN A PSYCHIATRIC UNIT AND HOW I MOVED ON

"Mental health problems don't define who you are. They are something you experience. You walk in the rain and you feel the rain, but, importantly, YOU ARE NOT THE RAIN."

—Matt Haig

O ur stories make us who we are. Every single experience we have makes us who we are today. The good, the bad, and everything in between. You might be able to pinpoint certain experiences as turning points in your life, events that triggered a chain reaction that led you along a certain path. I know I certainly can. These pivotal points in our timelines are what we often focus on, and rightly so. These events are the ones embedded in our minds as the reasons our lives went down the right path, or the not-so-right one. These defining points in our lives are often the reason to explain why we are the way we are. I'm going to share some of my triggers with you, and maybe you'll be able to see each red flag along the way, both the ones I missed and the ones I noticed. It is no secret that my life has been a series of unfortunate events. But alongside these events have been some good ones too. And I find that often the good things get overlooked by the bad. Everybody does it. The good things become overshadowed by some poor stroke of luck that we faced around the same time.

Here's a tidbit about me… throughout my life I have worn a great many different hats, taking on different roles, as we all do. The hat analogy works well for me. It is something I grasped a hold of when trying to explain who I am and who I have been. Allow me to share with you another poem, one which gives you an overview of both who I am and what I've done with my life. I will, of course, go into more detail in the rest of this chapter, but for me, this is just the perfect way to share with you who I am.

I Love Wearing Hats

I love wearing hats. My head is used to being covered by hats.
My head has donned many, many hats for years.
The wife hat had been on my head for almost 30 years.
My beautiful mom hat had been part of my outfit for almost 28 years.
I was a proud, confident medical professional hat wearer for 31 years.
The assortment of hats did not stop there. I also wore various other hats such as
bible study leader, close friend, neighbor, sister, and daughter, to name a few.
Things have changed though.
My head has been bare for months and months now. I don't know who I am without my hats.
I moved to Arizona and a big dilemma came to my mind.
How do I travel up and down the streets of Arizona without anything on my head?
Who I am if I don't have my mom hat or professional hat on?
Five years ago, I suffered through a terrible divorce. One by one, I lost my array of hats.
What was once a staple in my ensemble was now an item I struggled to even locate. CHANGE
I took my roles/ my hats for granted. I never realized how much of me was associated
with the hats I was wearing. I had dreamt of being a mom since I was a little girl
lining up my dolls on my bedroom's windowsill, readying them all for a dinner
of Kool-Aid and cookies. I had visions of working at a hospital with a white lab
coat and helping patients as they desperately needed my help to feel better.
I longed for the desire to find me again. I wanted so badly to want to
be a part of something again. I wanted to wear hats again.

After years of struggling, I found the courage for a fresh start and my road took
me to Arizona. I had no idea what God had for me here in the desert.
My children were all living their lives and doing well in the Midwest and the East Coast.
I was searching without family or friends, far from all that I had known.
I left a job that I had loved, but couldn't seem to find the right fit here in the desert.
I wasn't sure where I was to turn.
I wasn't sure what I was supposed to be doing.
Was I even where God wanted me to be? Dear Lord, please give me a hat.
I wanted assurance; I needed assurance, but what I got was so very unexpected.
What I received was a time of respite, a time of reflection.
God had landed me in a "hat free zone" for now.

The desert is not what I had expected, but it has given me so much more.
I'm trying on a few hats from time to time—author and
speaker hat, volunteer hat, and part time job
hat—but for now the only hat that I seem to need is "Child of God" hat.

———————

I'm sure I'm not the only woman, the only person, who has felt the same way. You split yourself between the different roles in your life, donning a different persona as needed. The warm loving mother, the hard-working professional, the reliable friend, and the list goes on. It can be exhausting to say the least, but nothing is more confusing than going from having all these different hats to having none at all. It can be hard to know who you truly are without the identity associated with your different roles. Learning to be who you are is difficult, but getting to know yourself is a gift. I encourage you to think back on your life, whether you're in your twenties or in your eighties, and think about all the different hats you've worn. I bet you'll be shocked by how many hats have graced your head.

Write a few sentences about the hats you've worn or the hats you'd like to wear.

_____

_____

_____

_____

_____

_____

x x x x x

I NEVER KNEW I
WAS DIFFERENT

This is the first thought to cross my mind as I begin to share my story with you. The simple fact of the matter was that I had quite literally no idea I was any different from the kids around me when I was young. My story begins in Texas. I was born on a hot June day in 1962. I was the first-born child to my parents. My first breaths were taken in Corpus Christi, Texas. This would be one of the few places I traveled through in life. I don't really remember my time there. I was young when my mother moved to Minnesota, with both me and my little sister in tow.

For the first three years of my life I was part of a three-person family: my mom, my dad, and me. December 1965, my world was changed forever. Remember what I said about trigger moments in our lives? Well this was the catalyst that pushed my life along a different path. Infidelity touched our family and my father left.

My mother was pregnant with my little sister at the time my father left us. Soon after he left, my little sister was born in Corpus Christi. We still lived there at this point. My dad visited us from time to time, and I had to go out with him and his girlfriend. Even at four years old that wasn't my idea of fun. Children know a lot more than we give them credit for, believe me. After the divorce, not too long after my sister was born, my mom made the decision to move us to Minnesota, where my grandparents lived. With a young child, a baby, and two suitcases in hand, my mother traveled alone to move in with my grandparents in their small apartment—the apartment which would become the first home I could properly remember.

One memory that is clear in my mind, and probably one of my earliest proper memories, not one of those hand-me-down memories that you feel like you remember because people tell you about it, was my first Christmas in Minnesota. My grandfather bought a Christmas tree that was too tall for our little apartment, so he cut off the very top and covered it in aluminum foil. We then put sparkly lights, homemade ornaments of construction paper links, and candy canes on the tree. As a child, I thought my aluminum-foil-topped tree was the most beautiful tree I had seen. My grandparents' apartment was cramped, with three adults and two children; we were under each other's feet constantly. But in the best way imaginable. This was what family felt like to me. The closeness, the love, the memories, it felt right to me, at my young, impressionable age.

For years after that Christmas, I began to draw and write short stories about my experiences growing up. One such extract belongs right here. This is something so close to my heart; it makes me ache with feelings, even now. I am proud of my mother. To think of her uprooting everything with two young children and moving cross-country. I can't quite imagine how she must have felt. But she did it for us, my sister and me. And, as a mother, that is something I am more than familiar with.

A Chocolate Girl Growing Up in a Blonde Minnesota World

———

I never realized I was different. Let me restate that—I never knew what different was until I was told I was not like the others. My mother moved to Minnesota from Texas alone and scared. Mother took a bus for over 20 hours, with two suitcases, a six-month-old and a four-year-old in tow. With no hands free and no one to help, she pushed through to get to her parents living in Minnesota. My grandparents were just my Grandma/ Abuela and Grandpa/Abuelo to me, little did I know that they were proud Mexican migrants originally from Texas trying to make it in Minnesota with their children. My grandparents spoke English and Spanish and that was a valuable skill when working with the summer migrants that came up from Mexico each year to work the fields and harvest.

———

Write about your upbringing—your family, your home. Try to do it in only a few lines. The very basic outline of your childhood.

_____

_____

_____

_____

_____

The next year passes in a state of childhood bliss. You know how it is before life gets too complicated. Days of happiness, love and family surrounding you. Before you venture out into the wider world you are safe in your little bubble, away from the influences of other people, of society. This is the time before you know truly what the world around you is like. You only really have your own family to compare yourself to, and because you are family, and you are young, chances are that you will be very similar people. After all, your family are the ones raising you.

In September 1967, I started kindergarten. A huge part of our lives, even though we might not remember the exact nature of the time we spend there, it comes in feelings and flashes. Maybe you remember specific events that happened to you at this time in your life, maybe you don't. For me, what I do remember is how proud I felt on my first day of kindergarten, when my mother took me to school. My mother was strong, confident, and beautiful, and I was so proud to be her daughter. I wanted to show her off to all the other children. But that day, something changed in me. A switch was turned, something that I now can never take back, something which fills me with embarrassment and sadness. All the other children had two parents take them to school. It used to make me feel so guilty until I came to the realization that I was just a little girl. I was a child just trying my best, and I didn't know any better. Children have this intrinsic need to fit in, something that I struggled with throughout the rest of my school career, if you can call it that!

After my mother took me on my first day of kindergarten, my grandfather, my abuelo, took on the role. He donned the hat of the one in charge of my walk to school each day. From the second day of kindergarten all the way through third grade this caused me to feel ashamed and embarrassed. I made my abuelo walk a full block behind me because I was embarrassed of him. His accent, his skin color, the fact that he was so different from the other parents dropping their kids off at school. It brought an attention to me that I didn't want to deal with. When I think back now about what that must have felt like for him, I can't even begin to understand. But each day he walked me to school a block behind, without protest or argument, making sure I got there safely. I share this with you so that you understand my life, without censoring who I was and who I am. There's no need for judgment; what I want to say is that everybody makes mistakes, makes decisions that hurt other people. By sharing my own with you, maybe you'll be able to admit to your own. Maybe you'll be able to forgive yourself, and I hope that you can. We are human, at the end of the day. We are flawed and fragile; we are allowed to mess up. Remember that, it's important.

"Mistakes are always forgivable if one has the courage to admit them."

—Bruce Lee

What do you think about this quote?

_____

_____

_____

_____

_____

In August 1970, I started Catholic school. This was something entirely alien for me. Not only was I petrified of the nuns (they still scare me!) but we had to wear uniforms too. The uniforms, meant to put us all on an even keel, made me stand out from the crowd. My skin color was different from the rest of the girls in my class. Very different. Before, it had been obvious, thanks to my abuelo when he walked me to school, but at Catholic school the distinction between me and the rest of the girls was stark. So very, very obvious. If you've never been in a room full of people who look completely different from yourself then you'll not know how it truly feels. It made me feel hot and cold at the same time. Embarrassed but protective.

Instead of owning my differences, which is what I would encourage anybody out there to do, I tried to bend myself to fit in with the rest of the girls. A square peg in a round hole springs to mind. There was so much kneeling, so much shame and guilt. It wasn't a happy time in my life. Not all Catholic schools are like this, I'm sure. Remember that this was many decades ago too! Things have (hopefully) changed a lot since then. But this atmosphere of fear, shame, and guilt was not conducive to good mental health, let me tell you. This is the first time I am called "spic" by kids on the playground. Never had I imagined that a simple label could be hurled as an insult. A fact, twisted to hurt. Up until this time, the worst name I had been called was "dodo brain" or "poopy head." Still, at this age I didn't quite understand what it meant to be different. Not yet. That would come later.

In June of 1971, my mom bought a new house. I told you she was a strong, independent woman! She was somebody to look up to. With two kids and a rocky history, she built herself back up and bought her own house. This brought a great deal of mixed feelings. It meant no longer living with my grandparents, whom I loved dearly, behind closed doors. But I was also excited for the separation from them. Across the street from our new home was a wooded area. Dense and thick trees clustered together. Overwhelmed with a new house, a new neighborhood, and no longer having my grandparents near, I decided in the infinite wisdom of an almost ten-year-old that I would live there instead. In the woods, alone. I think all children try to run away at some point in their lives; it feels like a rite of passage to me! I ran away for a grand total of three hours before returning home. I decided that I liked the new house and could manage without seeing my grandparents every day. It's crazy what a little bit of darkness and cold temperatures can do to your decision-making skills! Three hours felt like an eternity!

My mom moved us in with her new husband in June 1974, three years after we moved into our new home. They had dated for three years, so it wasn't quick by any means. It was a change that took some getting used to for my sister and me. One change was now there was a man in this house full of estrogen. Another big change for us here was that moving also meant moving to a new school. In August 1974, I graced the halls of a new school as the new girl. When you're new to a school, you're like a commodity. Everybody wants to know the new girl. For the first time in my life I experienced how it felt to be the center of attention.

A year later and I was ready to start junior high school. With a relatively easy year of schooling under my belt, I was thrown in the deep end when I started my new school. The teasing started pretty much straight away. I had long, dark hair and brown skin. All the other girls were white and mostly blonde. The difference is very apparent when you're already at that awkward preteen phase of your life, when you don't quite feel like a teenager or a child. The teasing continued, but some girls were kind to me too. At this point, I started that strange phase of developing. My body changed shape in a way that the girls around me didn't. I was ahead of the curve, so to speak. Something else to make me stand out. It was just what I needed! Boys began to give me attention thanks to my developing curves. This was attention I was not comfortable with.

Over the next year or so I become more aware of my own body than I've ever been. I find myself so self-conscious, not only for my skin tone, although that is still a significant part of it, but because I bloomed in ways the other girls hadn't yet. I found myself comparing my figure to theirs, dying to see somebody else's body doing the same thing as mine. Sleepovers were the very bane of my existence, as you can imagine! As were the school showers after physical education. Those showers! Is there anything else that could possibly make a young man or woman feel more sensitive about their bodies than those showers?! I think not! My body felt uncomfortable. Like it didn't belong to me. I wanted the slim, straight up and down figures of the other girls.

Where junior high school was bad, high school was of course worse. All of those raging hormones trapped in such a small space makes for an uncomfortable experience for even the most "typical"-looking person. I'm convinced that even the popular kids don't like high school. Navigating all those social situations while your body is making your life difficult too is just a cruel twist of fate. My sympathy goes out to every kid in high school. I wouldn't go back there for the world!

The second I walked through those double-glass doors to the high school in August 1976, I realized that I was one of very few girls with breasts in my grade, the only one with boobs, hips, and thighs. An adult body trapped alongside the mind of a teenager. An adult body in a sea of flat chests and hipless figures. The attention I received for my curves went beyond being just uncomfortable. It was lude and rude and made me hate myself even more than I already did. Couple that with my dark skin, eyes, and hair, and it was true self-hatred! In my small town, there were very, very few people of color in my high school, never mind another Mexican. I coped the best I could, mostly by ignoring the comments, stares, and bullying. I brushed it all under the rug and pretended that I was just like the other girls. I wasn't fooling anybody of course; a brown girl stands out like a, well, like a brown girl in a sea of while girls. I was pretty hard to miss.

✖ ✖ ✖ ✖ ✖

BLOSSOMING AND BLOOMING

Things began to change again when I was invited to my first dance in October 1976. Having been at the school a couple of months, I'd managed to fall into a routine of straight-up denial that I was any different from the other girls. I was happy to be asked to the dance. It felt grown-up, exciting even. When I asked my mother if I could go, she said no. I was heartbroken. I didn't understand. When I asked why, she said it was because I would get pregnant. That was the reason. Yes, you read that right. Getting pregnant seemed to be in the Mexican mother's handbook of fears for their daughters, no matter where you lived. She was trying to protect me in the best way she could. But the decision to not let me go to the dance triggered something within me. Another catalyst, or turning point, if you will. I did want to be seen in any sexual manner. My attention shifted from my boobs and hips and my skin color to my weight. I began to watch everything I ate, focusing with tunnel vision on calories and my intake. I joined the track team to run off the excess, not because I liked to run but because I wanted to keep my weight down and decrease my breasts and hips. It became an obsession very quickly. It was one of the only things I was able to control. I could control what I ate, what exercise I did. In a world where I had little control, this became the center of everything. The American Psychiatric Association defines eating disorders as, "illnesses in which the people experience severe disturbances in their eating behaviors and related thoughts and emotions. People with eating disorders typically become pre-occupied with food and their body weight..."

Do you have anything you'd consider to be an obsession? Is it healthy or unhealthy?

_____

_____

_____

_____

_____

_____

In February 1977, the next social event on the school calendar came barreling at me, full throttle—the Sadie Hawkins dance— which basically means that the girl has to ask the guy. One of my best friends was a guy, somebody I hung out with all the time. I wanted to ask him to the dance. After the last fiasco, I decided to do so without asking for my mom's permission. I was fairly certain he'd say yes. I'd been getting those kinds of vibes from him for a while. But when I asked him I was left heartbroken yet again, not for the reasons you would have presumed. No, instead of him saying no because he wasn't interested in me, he said no because his mom said he wasn't allowed to date a Mexican. It turned out he did actually like me and wanted to go with me to the dance, really badly. Something as nominal as the color of my skin prevented him from saying yes. As you can imagine, this didn't do much for my confidence.

Throughout the rest of that year, I found myself having to adapt who I was in order to fit in. I'd try to hide my ever-blossoming figure. I tried so hard no to attract attention to myself, preferring to stay with my tight-knit group of friends. Wallflower comes to mind as my goal during this time. Something I remember vividly, which I'm sure some of you ladies out there have experienced as well, is the experience of running track when you have quite large breasts. It's a chore, let me tell you! Wrapping my breasts in ACE bandages and wearing two bras to hide my chest was a daily occurrence. And it can bring a lot of unwanted attention, especially if you're trying to hide in the shadows like I was. As much as I tried to hide myself away, blending into the many faces of the other girls in my class, an older boy took a shine to me. He noticed me after track practice and came over to say hello. We became friends. We could talk for hours, and he could make me laugh. I began to beg my mother to let me date him. After months, she finally relented. He treated me well and seemed to like me for me with no hidden agenda. To this date, I am grateful for that. However, it was hard for me to ignore the jeers from his friends when he wasn't around: "I'd never be caught dead dating a 'spic.'" Those words, and the venom behind them, are forever engraved in my mind. Strangely, that wasn't the reason we broke up. He never knew of those unkind words, nor ever thought of me that way. I managed to put on a brave face and ignore the blatant racism from others. My mother's constant worry and strictness was difficult to overcome and led us to break up. He was a nice guy and I was absolutely crushed.

That Thanksgiving and Christmas break, I spent the whole holidays hiding away at home. I felt absolutely broken from the break-up, possibly more so than a typical teenager would, but I didn't know any different back then. My bed was a safe haven from any potentially embarrassing or upsetting situations. I didn't go to any parties or see my friends. I think often the power of our bed is underestimated. It was the only place I felt calm, complete, and normal-ish. By January 1978, I tried my best to leave my bed and pulled myself together enough to put myself out into the world again. I still shied away from accepting my differences from the other girls and did my very best to pretend I was the same as they were. During this time, I began dating again, very aware that, despite my different skin color and figure, boys were certainly very interested in me. Unfortunately, boys were a little too interested in sex for a Catholic girl like me. I said, "No thank you!" to that and walked away. The stress of my body, my skin, my mother, and just school all seemed to be too much to handle.

It was around this time that I had my first suicidal ideation. I dreamed of what the world would be like if I didn't exist. In my mind, it would be a better place. I'd remove much of the burden from those around me. The following is a poem about this time in my life.

Take Away the Pain

It's funny. I have always thought of myself as a well-balanced, funny, kind person. I had no idea there was really another "Me" that was not so kind or funny and definitely not well balanced.

Where does the funny one go? Does it just die for a while? Does it ever come back? Or does it need to be reinvented every single time there is pain? I will take the challenge/journey of investigating the where's and what if's of losing oneself to pain and how all that can have a major effect on how you live your life. Or if you choose to live your life.

When I was much younger, maybe first or second grade, I remember sitting in my grandmother's cushy crotcheting chair in her apartment and thinking, "How come I'm not outside playing with friends?" "Why am I tired?" "Why does my little sister cry so much?" The answers always seem to be just beyond my reach.

"Am I failing?" "Am I not being the perfect, quiet little girl I am expected to be?" There was nothing worse in my mind than not fulfilling my role of "good little girl," "perfect little girl." Who had to have her tights match her skirt, which matched her shoes?

Who never caused a fuss to prevent mom from yelling or hitting?

I had a job to do. It was my responsibility. If I didn't do my job, everything would fall apart.

My first suicide ideation occurred when I was 15 years old. My mother had a very difficult time allowing me to date or go out with boys even in groups of boys and girls. My mother had to know where I was going, who I was going with, how I was getting there, and what I was wearing. I remember a Saturday night in May, putting on a new outfit to head out with friends to a movie. I felt incredible. My hair was long and straight and had no static for once. My Calvin Klein jeans fit just tight enough, flowered halter top, and I had on my irresistible Bonne Bell Bubble Gum lip gloss.

I walked out of my room only to be faced with the backhand of my mother. She ripped my halter top off of me saying I looked like a tramp and that was exactly the kind of girl she knew I would turn out to be. I was stunned. Nothing had been showing, all the important parts were covered up, yet it was not good enough once again. She told me I was not going out and that I had better break up with "that older, no good football player," Devastated didn't even cover half of what I was feeling. Here is a woman that says she loves me more than anything else, but she hits me and calls me names. What was wrong with me? Why couldn't I just do things right for once? I hated upsetting her. I needed to do better; I had to do better. But could I do better?

The resounding answer that pounded in my brain was "no." She was absolutely right. I was no good. I couldn't do anything right. I couldn't do things like I was supposed to. Why would God make me this way? Why couldn't I understand and do all that she wanted?

I had to ease her pain. I had to make my pain stop.

My mom would feel so much better if she didn't have to deal with a kid like me. She deserved so much better. She was a divorced mom doing the best she could, and again, I was causing her trouble, causing her pain.

I knew there were bottles of pills in my parents' medicine cabinet. Could I be brave enough, smart enough to actually make my mom happy with this deed? This removal of me to make her life easier?

By June 1978, I was running or biking five miles every single day trying my very best to lose my hips and breasts. This became the very focus on each of my days. I had to exercise to the extreme. It felt like such a high, a sense of control that no one else could stop. I didn't know this was indicative of something more sinister; I was only a young girl and eating disorders were not spoken about back then. It seemed to be this nasty secret I held so very close to me. Eating disorders were barely even whispered about. So I thought that all this exercise was normal because I was only trying to achieve something all the other girls had. Then I started purging. Everything I ate I purged, it was the most effective way for me to lose weight and control part of my life when all else felt out of control. I ate at my mom's restaurant in order to try not to draw attention to my weight loss. Deep down, at this point, I think I knew that something was wrong. When I was purging it felt shameful and I knew it was something to be hidden. But that didn't stop me from doing it. If anything, as I saw myself making progress, losing weight, I saw this as a reason to carry on. I know I'm not the only one out there who has ever felt like this. So many of you will have sadly experienced the same.

In the midst of all the exercising, purging, and obsessing over my body, I added burning and cutting, or self-injury, to my list of harming myself. I also began dating my first serious boyfriend. We began to date in September 1979. I thought he was absolutely perfect, and in many ways he was. He loved me and supported me, and at that age, that felt incredible. It felt mature and right. My self-esteem slowly began to improve for the first time during this relationship and symptoms slowly declined. I saw myself in a much clearer light. That was until his mother told me, "No son of mine will ever marry a Mexican girl." All the hard work I'd put into overcoming my eating disorder and improving my self-esteem was ruined in those few words. My eating disorder, not that I knew that's what it was, worsened tenfold. Despite the cruel words from his mother, I carried on dating my boyfriend at the time. The relationship was serious, particularly for a teenager. We dated through graduation and beyond. The boyfriend that I first mentioned, the older guy who introduced himself while I was running track, came back into the picture for a short while during the summer break before college. We went out on a platonic "date," although it wasn't a date at all. We both knew that. It was two friends hanging out. We went to the beach and had dinner. Old feelings began to arise within me, I'm not ashamed to admit. We all hold a torch or sorts for the first person we dated, even if the flame is the size of a quarter. As it turned out, our feelings were soon dashed (because they weren't just on my part) when he found out I was in love with my boyfriend. He too was dating another girl anyway. We parted ways as friends and I was happy to return back to my boyfriend whom I loved dearly.

Starting college is a huge life event for anybody, and I was so excited to be a college girl. My freshman year was full of the normal college stuff—drinking, partying, attending classes, and meeting new people. Alongside that, I also visited my boyfriend at his college. We were still going strong. That didn't stop me from purging everything I ate. Because of the partying, I failed to get into the nursing program I so badly wanted to attend. Again, I was crushed, but I transferred to a community college. I carried on with my college education until June 1982, when I graduated and got ready to transfer to a larger university. All the while feeling so in control while I was now taking diuretics and laxatives to purge due to my busy schedule. It was at this point that I broke up with my boyfriend. He'd been my rock for so long, and it was a steep learning curve relearning how to be single after so long.

x x x x x

A FREEFALL INTO ADULTHOOD

Surprisingly, the stress and busyness of university decreased my eating disorders somewhat, but instead excessive drinking was used to numb the pain and stress. Studying and dating also began to take a large portion of my life. Both of these had a huge impact on my self-esteem. It began to slowly increase again, something I desperately needed. The university was slightly more diverse than my high school too, which also helped. Plus, by this stage, most women had developed their bodies, and I wasn't the only one with hips and breasts. I also found other women who knew the same secret and participated in the same-binge purge, laxative and diuretics, extreme exercise- web of lies. I found them in a support group on campus that saved my life. They understood like no one in my life ever had. In October 1985, I graduated from college with a degree in therapeutic recreation, which qualified me to be a Certified Therapeutic Recreation Specialist (CTRS), a job I was looking forward to sinking my teeth into. A CTRS organizes and leads interventions for people with disabilities, illnesses, or injuries to help improve their function through recreation and leisure. My practice focused almost exclusively on mental illnesses. During this time, my eating disorder had all but vanished. I had done my best to eat and exercise normally. Leading my clients to healthy well-being helped me as well. I also talked to a counselor and continued attending eating disorder support groups. They helped me feel good about myself. I truly tried to live the best version of my life.

Around this time, I also met my future husband. We married as college sweethearts in June 1986. It was a lovely day, filled with friends and family. I felt beautiful and happy, excited for the rest of my life. I couldn't wait to see what my husband and I would achieve together. A couple of months after the wedding, while we were still in that honeymoon period you hear about, we moved to Montana, away from family and friends. At the time, I did it because I loved my husband and I would have followed him anywhere. It didn't take me long to realize that jealousy and a lack of trust would appear in our marriage. He was new to marriage, just as I was, so compromise and learning to respect each other was its own journey.

During this time in my life, I faced a great deal of racism. The racism in Montana was like nothing I'd experienced yet, and I'd experienced more than my fair share already. Where the racism in Minnesota was more whispered and somewhat subtle, in Montana it felt more blatant and accepted. At my job as a recreational therapist, people would ask not to work with the "native girl," due to the color of my skin. This happened so regularly that I began to hate my job. I hated the treatment I faced and the fact that it was deemed appropriate to ask for me not to work with a patient who didn't like the color of my skin. After a lot of begging and pleading, my husband acquiesced and allowed us to move back home to Minnesota so that we could both attend graduate school. It was far more my idea than his, but he went along with it, which I was grateful for. By June 1989, we had both graduated and secured new jobs. Life was beginning to look up for us. And with the birth of our first child, the greatest achievement in my life thus far, I felt complete. My baby boy was born in March 1990. I'd wanted to be a mom all of my life, and when he arrived, I'd never felt more at home in myself and my role as mother. My husband and I were loving our roles as parents, and we were in the groove as husband and wife as well. When my daughter arrived just over two years later, in June 1992, I was so thrilled to add to our little family.

As some of you parents out there know, having a baby is not always as you'd expect it to be. Even with your second baby, things don't necessarily go as you envisioned they would. I loved my daughter so much, but the aftermath of the birth was not exactly as I hoped. She had terrible colic, which made life so much more difficult (as those out there with colicky babies know). This triggered the depression and anxiety that had always festered inside of me. I'd experienced bouts of depression and anxiety throughout my life, as you'll be able to tell from my story so far, but this was something more than I'd ever suffered with before.

You might be aware that often depression and anxiety go hand in hand. However, they are two very different things. Just to make sure we're all on the same page, let's take a look at the definitions of both.

The American Psychiatric Association defines depression as, *"Depression (major depressive disorder) is a common and serious medical illness that negatively affects how you feel, the way you think and how you act. Fortunately, it is also treatable. Depression causes feelings of sadness and/or a loss of interest in activities once enjoyed. It can lead to a variety of emotional and physical problems and can decrease a person's ability to function at work and at home."*[2]

Anxiety disorders are defined as, *"Anxiety is a normal reaction to stress and can be beneficial in some situations. It can alert us to dangers and help us prepare and pay attention… Anxiety disorders differ from normal feelings of nervousness or anxiousness and involve excessive fear or anxiety."* You can see how the two would sit hand in hand, feeding off one another. Lucky for me, I was one of the many people who experienced both!

Life was really hard for a while. I started Occupational Therapy school in August of that year. It felt manageable, as it was every other weekend. This, I hoped, would give me a chance to be a mother to two young children as well as work on my career. On the weekends, when I wasn't in school, I worked on a locked psychiatric unit at a major university hospital. This was a world

---

2 "Help with Depression," American Psychiatric Association, accessed February 28, 2021, https://www.psychiatry.org/patients-families/depression.

I'd never been privy to before. It's not like it is in the movies. It's raw and unfiltered, yet open and kind to helping those in need. I'm so thankful those units exist. The fact that the people on the units had fallen so low made me grateful for my own struggles.

During this time, my mental health began a steady decline. The workload, I believe, was the trigger. The balance of school, work, having two children under the age of three, depression, anxiety, and stress plunged me into a state of constant struggle. I felt like I was swimming against a roaring tide, never quite managing to catch my breath or to be the person I wanted to be. By January 1993, I decided to start seeing a therapist. I couldn't make my life work. I couldn't balance everything. I felt like the spinning plates I tried so desperately to keep in the air, were crashing to the ground. Shattered pieces seemed all around me. I was diagnosed with seasonal affective disorder, which meant that gray skies were my enemy. The American Psychiatric Association defines it as follows: "Seasonal affective disorder is a form of depression also known as SAD, seasonal depression or winter depression. People with SAD experience mood changes and symptoms similar to depression. The symptoms usually occur during the fall and winter months when there is less sunlight and usually improve with the arrival of spring... SAD is more than just "winter blues." The symptoms can be distressing and overwhelming and can interfere with daily functioning. However, it can be treated."[3]

3 "Seasonal Affective Disorder," American Psychiatric Association, accessed February 28, 2021, https://www.psychiatry.org/patients-families/depression/seasonal-affective-disorder

While my winter months were filled with sadness and depression, as the weather began to brighten up, so did my mood, which, to me at least, confirmed the diagnosis of SAD (an oddly fitting name, I know!).

Describe how each season makes you feel:

Spring

_____

_____

Summer

_____

_____

Fall

_____

_____

Winter

_____

_____

August 1993 was filled with sunshine! Literally and figuratively. I volunteered with the homeless and mentally ill and continued to work on psychiatric units. I began to fall back in love with my work and career. My job took me to locked inpatient adult units, locked inpatient adolescent units, and locked inpatient eating disorder units. I was able to throw myself into my work, and I felt that I was making a difference. The following year, with my children in preschool and my husband helping me more with the parenting and housekeeping, I began my internships for my degree in occupational therapy. Occupational therapists (or OTs) help people overcome any struggles caused by illness, aging, or accident in order for them to be able to carry out activities of daily living. They consider all aspects of a patient's need, including physical, psychological, social, and environmental. For me the focus would be on, you guessed it, mental illness, in order to allow people to live the best life they can. It was something that I'd seen myself doing since I started university, and I was so excited to begin my internships in pediatrics, neurology, orthopedics, and mental health in a women's prison. Through my internships, I learned so much about myself. I was able to compartmentalize, looking beyond my own worries and troubles. Seeing what my clients and patients were going through made me look at my own life. The things I saw and the stories I was told made me take a step back. I couldn't help but think, if my life had played out differently I could have been in their position, as could any of us. It doesn't take a lot for our lives to take a turn in ways we could never imagine. That's something I think a lot of people tend to forget. As Aaron Klug said, "You can't plan for the unexpected."

Have you ever had anything completely unexpected happen to you?

_____

_____

_____

_____

During August 1995 I finally graduated with my occupational therapy degree. I began working with a school district. My own children were doing well in all areas; they were the brightest spots in my own life. I continued seeing a therapist and eventually recognized that my own disordered thinking was a thing of the past, but my perfectionism still lingered. Like the smell of an awful fish! I decided that only I could make a choice to be stronger. I took life one day at a time, taking each day for what it was. Just one day ahead of me. My life continued on, as life tends to do, the following year. My children continued to do well in school, and I started working at a hospital in neurology, pediatrics, and eating disorders. While I loved my work, I soon realized that there was no way I could possibly give my all to my job and give my all to my family. Those feelings of inadequacy and unworthiness that I felt in the past began to rear its ugly head. I felt deep down inside me that I wasn't good enough. Couple this with my SAD, which came back each year with force during fall and winter. Not only that, but I so badly wanted another baby. I longed for it more than anything in the world. My husband disagreed, and that caused a rift in our marriage.

To try to alleviate the symptoms of SAD, as a family we traveled through the winter. While it helped for a time, depression spread throughout the rest of the year. This is when I began to take medication for depression and anxiety. Between 1995 and 1998, life carried on as normal. I coped as well as I could with the depression and anxiety, while struggling with feeling inadequate. Then, in February 1998, my life changed for the better yet again. My third child was born, and she quite literally saved my life, no exaggeration at all. I was so ill with depression and feeling the wrath of perfectionism that I had no idea what my life would be. Then my daughter came along and my other children loved her so much. I felt like I had something to look forward to yet again. This filled me with a glee and made it easier to cope with the depression and anxiety.

Fast forward over the next few years and my family and I carried on like any family. As a parent, my life was all kids—sports, travel, grades, friends, and church. The church became my community, our community, a space for my husband and children to feel alive and part of something bigger. Together, we went on mission trips all over the world—to the hills of Appalachia, the border towns of Mexico, and orphanages in Jamaica, to name a few—on missions to help make life better for others. As a family, we experienced so many incredible things and I am so grateful for this time in our lives. It was the part of our history where things just seemed to work. Then, in July 2008, things changed for the worst. The recession hit us as it hit many families. My husband's job was hit in a major way. The stress took its toll on

our marriage; decreased income, job changes, and economic uncertainty have a funny way of making life difficult! My husband
changed during this time. He became angry and bitter. He flirt-
ed with other women in a way he never had before. It made me
uncomfortable. It made me hate our relationship. That August,
we sold our dream home. The stress of so many changes was
enough to break even the most stable of relationships. And my
relationship with my husband was already rocky, so life became
difficult. We stayed together for probably longer than we should
have, only laughing together when we were on mini-vacations.
The rest of the time we were both left unfulfilled.

My older children continued to do well in their lives, busy
with high school and college, their friends, and their own lives.
Seeing them happy made me happy. My youngest bore the
brunt of the marital struggles. She saw our unhappiness in a
way I wish I could have shielded her from. It broke my heart
that she had to see her mom and dad so broken. After years
of difficulties, and hints of infidelity, my heart was completely
broken and the trust had gone. I had nothing left to give to the
relationship, and neither did my husband, and so we decided to
separate. The divorce became final in December 2012, just in
time for the holidays! Merry Christmas to me. I worried all the
time about whether my children would ever be okay again after
their parents divorced. My oldest found it difficult but took on
a parental role. He worried and cared about both me and his
dad, wishing for us to be okay. My middle child seemed angry
and this hurt me to the core. She struggled with the fact that we

weren't together anymore. My youngest was the most affected, of course. She seemed lost and scared. This was a horrific thing to see. To think that your actions have hurt your children is the worst feeling in the world for a parent. The worst. The pain never fully goes away.

My divorce left me feeling entirely inadequate. I felt like I'd failed at the one thing in life everybody should be able to do. My marriage had failed. I had failed. It was an awful feeling that pooled in the lowest pits of my stomach and left me feeling dread about what could come next.

Can you think about a time when you felt this way?

_____

_____

_____

_____

✗ ✗ ✗ ✗ ✗

THE LOWEST OF THE LOW: MY ROCK BOTTOM

By February 2013, I felt myself starting to pull the pieces of my life back together. I began to date more, after merely testing the waters during my separation. My fear and apprehension got in the way of anything fruitful. I was naive to say the least, after being married for most of my adult life, and when I met a man who was kind to me, I took that to mean love. We dated for more than a year while I struggled with depression, but I managed to hold things together for my children rather than anything else. When he proposed, I said yes. I was still on the rebound from my marriage, and it didn't take long for us to realize that it didn't feel right and we were rushing into things for the wrong reasons. The overwhelming feeling I got at this time was that I wasn't good enough, again. That ugly monster reared its head and made me question everything about myself. It made me hate who I was. We called off the wedding at the end of July 2014. I then finally allowed thoughts of what happened with the divorce, loss, and the reality of being alone to set in. The darkness seemed to envelope everything about me, my life, and my future. I'd never felt so bleak in all my life.

The darkness that came to settle over my life felt like a black cloud of despair closing in on me. So this is what they mean when they say rock bottom. There was nowhere below me to fall; I had fallen to the dungeon of my life. I knew enough that something was very, very wrong and that I needed some kind of safety net. I thank God every day that I had the ability to speak to have spoken to my friends, rather cryptically I have to admit. But all the same, they knew exactly when to intervene. One day, I remember saying something along the lines of, "I don't want my kids to worry about me," or "My kids would be better off without me." That distorted thinking was their clue that I needed help, pronto. It was a warning sign that I didn't want to be around anymore to burden my children, and that I was likely considering taking my own life. My children were my everything, so if those words were leaving my lips, I was envisioning leaving as well. Like many people in similar situations, I'd toyed with the idea of suicide but never anything concrete, more along the lines of just making all the pain go away. This is when you think about ending your life rather than doing anything about it. My heart goes out to every single person out there who has ever felt this way. Not only is it absolutely terrifying, but it's also very isolating. It wasn't until August 11, 2014, that I said something that made my friends jump into action.

My friends said that I told them, "I hate having my kids worry. I hate being a burden and I just know they'd be better off without me." I have a vague recollection of saying this and I cannot tell you how grateful I am that my friends took me seriously. They are my own little superheroes, without the capes, tights, and masks, of course. Without them, who knows where I would be. I honestly don't. Within minutes of these words coming out of my mouth, I was bundled into a car and driven to the hospital for suicide intake.

Here is an interpretation of what intake was like for me during that time...

I Miss My Shoes

I miss my shoes. They take your shoes away before you are about to enter onto a locked psychiatric unit. My shoelaces cause a threat, I guess. Little do they know, I would not even have the energy to pull both my shoelaces out of my Converse tennis shoes.

Energy is in short supply when you are entering a psych unit. You don't have energy, you don't have desire; you just are. Months before my arrival to the psych unit, I had told my friends, "If I ever begin to speak about not wanting to worry my kids, or I hate to be a burden to my kids, anything at all about relieving my kids of pain or worry, that is a large waving, red flag that I am in trouble." You see my kids are my everything. Nothing in my life has ever meant more to me than my children. Being a mother had been my goal since I was a little girl. If that goal was to get clouded or diminished, we were in trouble; rather, I was in trouble.

The trouble trumpet sounded on August 11, 2013 when I spoke to my girlfriends of how much I hated worrying my children. I knew my kids were distracted by how down I was and I felt they really should no longer have their mother be the focus of their thoughts.

Less than twenty minutes later, my friends were at my home and driving me to a hospital.

Crying and irrational thinking consumed my talk on the way to the hospital. I rambled, I sobbed, and all the while my friends were silently praying, listening, and attempting to drive down the highway, never caring about any speed limit.

I remember thinking, if I could just open my door. I had no forecasting ability that I would be crushed by oncoming traffic or that my body would be a mangled mess due to the speed we were traveling in, I just wanted to leave, I just wanted to sleep.

It wasn't that I wanted to die, I just wanted to escape, and sleep seemed the best choice.

Sleep seemed to be the center of my thinking once I arrived at the hospital.

I was asked over and over "Do you want to hurt yourself?" "Do you want to die?" and the statement I used to use when working on psychiatric units: "Do you have a plan to harm yourself?"

You see, psychiatric units are not foreign to me. Not because I have ever been a patient on one but because I have worked in mental health for over twenty years. Locked adolescent inpatient units, adult inpatient and outpatient units, residential eating disorders units, mental health correctional units in a women's prison, and on and on, that is where I not only earned a living but where I had found one of my passions.

Going to school to be a Therapeutic Recreations Specialist, then later an Occupational Therapist, helping people find their way was what I was called to do. There is nothing that suits me as well as helping children with disabilities or people of all ages struggling with mental illness. Some people talk about having a career or a job, but I have always felt that the work I do has been a calling, and I really have no choice nor any desire to do anything else than to do the work I do.

Working on psychiatric units, you get used to the harsh clanging of the metal doors closing and locking behind you when you walk onto a unit or prison area. It becomes your way of life, like the sound of water running as you brush your teeth. You don't actually hear the water after a while; it is just the background noise as you complete your daily ritual.

Nothing struck me more abruptly than the clang of those same metal doors I just mentioned. My triage nurse in the ER took my shoes with laces, took my purse, and took my phone, and an orderly proceeded to escort me to the locked adult unit. *The orderly tried to make a passing conversation, but I was numb to the mumblings coming out of his mouth until he said one sentence that somehow woke me from my trance: "I am so glad you are here and you did not end up like Robin Williams did." "What?" I remember thinking. "Robin Williams? What in the world is he talking about and what happened to Robin Williams?" The buzzing of the door brought me from those thoughts to what was lying ahead for me.*

The buzzing of the door I was about to proceed through was startling, but I had heard it many times before on other units while working. When those doors closed shut, however, and the metal of the locks closed, it seemed to vibrate in my ears and it scared me to my core. Was this how loud it had been when I would walk patients through doors like these after escorting them from group sessions? Was this how scared they had been when they were told to follow therapists, nurses, doctors, and orderlies all day long through these same doors? How did I not realize this? How could I have been so insensitive?

My nurse introduced herself to me and explained that I would have to change clothes, and no I would not be getting my shoes back while in the unit. Why I was so obsessed with my shoes during this process, I have no idea, but I can only guess that they provided some sort of comfort, some sort of normalcy to me.

It was amazing to me what stood out during this process. I don't remember the activity room with the TV, or the patients sitting watching the TV, as I walked past coming onto the unit, nor did I seem to see the nurses' desk with the glass enclosure, but I do remember the dark blue booties with the nonslip bottoms and that I was to put on light blue scrubs to wear as my "patient uniform."

I was led to the room closest to the nurses' desk. As numb and distracted as I was at that time, I did know, however, that those patients on suicide watch or those with violent behavior were always housed next to the nurses' desk area. Guess where my room was located? Next to the nurses' desk. This would be my home for however long they felt was necessary.

I have always been pretty active and in good physical shape, however, on that day, I remember feeling like my feet were just too heavy to lift with each step I took. It was as if I was walking on the beach after a rain and wet sand surrounded my feet and I just could not seem to lift them to take my next steps. I shuffled to the activity room. My feet were not only heavy, but they stuck to the floor. Stupid nonslip bottoms! Did I mention that I missed my shoes, dang, can I just have my shoes? Who knows, they were probably full of imaginary sand as well.

A chair with brown and tan stripes was available next to a kind-looking black man staring off into the direction of the TV. Even as he stared off and never lost his focus, he said "I'm Emil. And don't let this place scare you. These folks will take good care of you. Don't you worry." His eyes never wavered from the TV. For a moment, I wasn't even sure he was speaking to me, but he slowly rose up and looked me straight in the eyes and said, "You are welcomed here." And he headed down the hallway of rooms.

Jeopardy was on the TV. Usually, I was up for a challenge with Mr. Trebek, but today, I didn't even know what day it was.

The orderly that had brought me to the unit asked if I had filled out my menu yet. "My menu? What menu? I have to eat? Wait, I have to DECIDE what to eat?" I began to cry. Obviously the choice of pasta or chicken was just too much for my brain to process at that moment. My nurse came from behind the nurses' desk and asked if I wanted to lie down before dinner and I replied, "I don't know. Am I tired?" Ok, a moment of background, I worked my way through high school, college, and graduate school, making decisions left and right, not always confident but definitely able to decipher whether I was tired or not!

I woke up to the sound of crashing. I came out of my room to see a "new girl" pulling down the dinner trays from the stacks of pasta and chicken for the patients. It took two orderlies and a nurse to calm the "new girl" down and lead her to MY ROOM!

"Um, excuse me," I thought to myself, "I am here to sleep. There is no way that loud, crash-causing disruptor of a girl is going to be in my room, is she?"

After dinner, I shuffled back to my room. In my room, just like all the other rooms on the unit, were two twin beds in a sterile, cold, gray cinder block walled room that had a single plastic chair at the edge of the far-left bed. One of the orderlies was sitting in the cold plastic chair as the "new girl" slept. It felt strange having someone in my room, having two someones in my room. I wanted to be alone, I needed to sleep.

I have always been an expert sleeper. Growing up, I loved being alone, and lying in bed was a great escape. An even greater escape was sleep. Living in Minnesota in the winter can be hard when it is gray skies and days of thirty below zero with an even lower wind chill. Wind on your face feels like sharp needles cutting into *your cheeks on days like that. So what do you do on freezing cold days? Easy choice for me; I lay on my bed, I write, I draw, I read, and most importantly, I listen to music. Music has always been a great companion to my solitude on my bed. Working every day at my mom's Mexican restaurant allowed me the opportunity to make money, and although I saved most of what I made, my weakness was albums. I had a great collection of music to meet every mood I was going through. As my journey took me through a new elementary school every few years then to middle school teasing and fringes of puberty, then on to womanhood, boys, and heartbreak in high school, music and my bed were my sole confidants and shoulders to lean on.*

I could easily fall asleep to Crosby, Stills, and Nash; Dan Fogelberg; The Eagles; or sprinklings of Elton John. I had been known to wake up hugging many albums as my comfort through the night. Sleep was my respite from a life of uncertainty. It was the one thing I could count on to help me deal with all that was unpredictable in my life.

Have you ever hit rock bottom? What did your rock bottom look like?

_____

_____

_____

_____

I'm not sure I can ever explain what it felt like to be on the other side of the locked doors of the psychiatric unit effectively. I'm going to try my best, but it's one of those things that, until you've experienced it yourself (and I hope you never do), you can't possibly imagine, to be submerged in this alternate reality, away from the real world and those you love. Let me say this,

I wouldn't swap getting admitted for the world. It saved me. It saved those around me. And for that, I can never express how grateful I am. The whole point of this book is to share with you what it was like to go from being a professional inside a psychiatric unit to a patient and beyond. As far as I'm aware, this is a pretty rare occurrence in the grand scheme of things. The best way I can share with you what it felt like is through poetry. Poetry is my saving grace, the way I can make sense of my experiences, emotions, and thoughts in a way that's cohesive. The following poems were written both right before, while I was in the psychiatric unit, and after my release. I'll warn you, they're not for the faint of heart and may seem pretty dark.

Dirty Windows

She stands at the window, no thought of a quick release
She knows why she is here, caught up in this hospital with freaks.
She is not like the others; she's so different, she has a clue.

She stands at the window, irritated by the view
Why can't they do anything right; why can't these windows be washed?
She has to be in here, this cage of snoops and rules so unfair
She tries to find release, but dirty windows is all they share

She stands at the window, feeling empty and unloved
Dirty windows, dirty past
Who would love a girl so ugly and untrue?

They won't listen, they just don't want to hear
She tries to tell them, she tries not to feel,
"Can't you see I'm hurting, can't you see the pain?"
but dirty windows is all they see, dirty windows
is all that's me.

Red Is Beauty

———————

I slice, I scratch, I burn and I pick
Red is my goal, my desire, my feel

I hold the pen in my right hand, ready to begin
The pain is so loud, so needy for release
I dig in my arm, no red to be seen
More force, more intent and the beauty begins to show.

My goal is to feel, to remember what it's like
My goal is the red, the color I adore.
It takes me away, away from the others
Red is my out, my chance to escape.

Pain has a voice, it is scarlet and it is red
My pain calls for assistance, for someone to help.
I won't let it be voiced, just too hard to explain
But my red is the beauty, the beauty of my pain.

Smells

———————

No other smell like it, it burns and it chars
The smell stays in your nostrils for days at a time

No other smell like it, the smell of skin singed and burned
The release of the emotion, the letting go of the hurt

No other smell like it, the smile begins to form
Finally a hope of release, release of the pain

No other smell like it, the scars seem to last
I know, more pain to come, more scars to be had

My secret release of the feelings, feelings so bad
No other smell like, so glad to have the burn.

No other smell like,
No pain like it too.

Can you write a poem about one of your own life events?

_____

_____

_____

_____

_____

_____

_____

_____

_____

_____

_____

_____

_____

_____

_____

_____

_____

Somewhat dark, I know! I wanted to share with you the rawness, the times when I hit rock bottom. They may not be pretty, but they're real. Let me give another shoutout to my friends and to God's prompting to reach out to them. While I was on the psychiatric unit, under suicide watch, my friends went to my home and got rid of my wedding dress and bridesmaid dresses. Cancelling the wedding had been one of the triggering factors in my mental health decline, for certain, and removing those reminders (something I couldn't bring myself to do) meant that I could return home to a blank slate. Not only did they do that, but they also cleaned my house from top to bottom and restocked the fridge for my return. How lucky am I to have people like that in my life? While I was on the unit, I lost my job. Because things were not bad enough, another layer was added to my depression cake. My employer wasn't too thrilled with the idea of hiring somebody with mental health issues, and when I finally returned home, I took the time to heal and see my therapist as often as I could. For the first time, my health was a priority. This next poem is dedicated to all the "givers" out there. I think this one will provide you with all the "feels."

Being Leftovers

Does it ever seem that no matter how much you do, there never seems to be enough?
Enough time. Enough money. Enough energy. Enough YOU.
You give and give to so many others that there is never enough for you.
You make sure everyone else has what they need, but you don't have what you need.
You may think IN TIME, I will meet my needs. In TIME, it will be my turn.
Friends need consoling, a shoulder to lean on, and you are glad to be there.
Kids need time and money. They need your help, and you're glad to do it.
Your job needs your very best to service the clients, complete the paperwork,
and help your coworkers, and of course you need that paycheck.
Your spouse needs laundry done, meals made, and a forever friend, of course.
It makes you feel good to be needed. It makes you feel good to be serving others.
When is it your TIME? When are your needs met? Aren't you tired of being leftovers?
When everyone has taken and you are left standing, what remains for you?
Is it always just leftovers?

I'm sure feeling like leftovers is nothing new to most of you reading this book. It took me reaching the lowest of the low points in my life to realize that I had to prioritize me. I was no good to anyone else if I didn't look after myself. This started with seeing my therapist and putting all of my strength into my recovery. I was determined to be able to function as I once had, granted with better self-care and a lot less stress. Strangely, I found that leaving the psychiatric unit was just as difficult for me as being admitted in the first place. This was something I sure hadn't anticipated. Another poem? Why not!

Shadows

Pulling toward the shadows.

The hairs on the back of my neck stood up. My skin began to crawl. I could feel their presence behind me. When I would look back, all I saw was darkness.

Was I willing to enter the darkness again? I had been down that trodden pathway too many times to count. This was the path not taken—well, not taken in many, many years.

Despite the eeriness of my skin's reaction and my hair being at attention, there was somehow a cruel deceiving welcoming. Like an abandoned home, never to be visited again.

What would it be like to "go home again"? What would it be like to revisit my youth?

They say, "you can't go home again," but is that really true? As I feel the darkness, the shadows approaching, there is a decision to be made. It could be so familiar, so comforting to just make a short visit. Just one last time. "For old times' sake," as they say. I have had this feeling before, I just never looked back. Have not looked back in years.

As I get a glance of the shadow, I am reminded not only of its comfort but also of the struggles that come along with it. The shadows don't just come once or twice, they arrive daily, maybe even an hourly occurrence forcing me to make a choice.

"Do I allow the light to diffuse the shadow's presence? Or do I turn away from The Light and allow the shadow to enter my dwelling?

I remember finding comfort in that cool, dark space. No one could see me. No one could find any light to reach out to. Did I want that again? Did I want the distance, the dark? Did I want the comfort of isolation and the lie of caring and warmth?

As I contemplate my dilemma, I see a flicker of radiance, a glimpse of the other side.

The light is trying to peek through. It is trying to make its presence known. Not in a bold way, but just a slow, familiar return. It is as if a dear friend slowly comes into the kitchen and that familiar sound of the screen door slamming behind. It somehow makes you smile.

You know why it's there. You know why this beautiful, loving light returns. It is truly comforting. Warm arms reach out to hold you, to let you know "I am here." It lets you know, it has always been there. You just needed to push away the shadows. You needed to release the ideal of your former self. You needed to ignore the mistaken appeal of control.

(John 1:5: The light shines in the darkness, and the darkness has not overcome it.)

The choice is mine, this an all too familiar choice. This "I thought I never had to worry or face this question ever again." Do I lose the shadow of my former self and expose the light into every tiny corner of my life? Or do I attempt to push away any light and return to the "what was" and the "could have been"?

That road of shadows is a tricky one. It deceives and lies to you. It tells you to try it, just one last time. You stop whenever you choose. The story sounds the same. It tells you you're not good enough, not nearly up to par.

Am I okay to be just as I am? I dreamed and I hoped for release from the dark.

Twenty years of recovery, some dark but mostly light. I can't give it up. I can't give up the light. I make the choice.

*I release the shadows and welcome my light. I need to remember
when bad times arrive that I have a choice and ask myself,
is recovery worth the risk? Today I choose no.*

*I need to remember that around every corner, within all my life; I need
to stand firm and make a choice just for me. I am worth it. I do deserve
health. There will always be shadows and always be trials. The memory
of recovery, the goodness of hope is what keeps me going day after day.
Goodbye to dark shadows; I will be okay. When I think I can't make it
and things are too hard, I'll remember that good times will come.*

I need to be patient and just hold on. Take a deep breath, then choices can be made.

Today my choice is me and I will not accept dark. I am worth it and I am enough.

———

**How does this personal account make you feel?
Have you ever experienced similar?**

_____

_____

_____

_____

_____

I have found that the "darkness" of your past is something that
tends to linger unless you address it. Even on your best days
you remember what it was like to feel the way you did back
then. But the feelings are removed, almost like they happened
to somebody else. The memory of the incident becomes like a
permanent scar, healed, but a reminder of what occurred. Even-

tually, we are able to come to terms with our behavior during these times. We acted through our mental illness, rather than our rational thinking. The suicidal thoughts were not me. They were my illness. This is something that I remind myself of every day, and will do for the rest of my life. Remember, you are not what you did when you were unwell. Yes, take ownership of your actions if they hurt others, but move the hell on. The past is the past and you can't change the things you did or the person you were. Focusing on the now, on the person you are now in this very moment, the person you wish to be in the future, that is what's going to help you to heal. I know it's difficult, but nothing in life worth having is easy.

✖ ✖ ✖ ✖ ✖

REBUILDING MY LIFE

When I left the unit and returned back to my home, which my friends had made absolutely perfect for me, I buckled down and saw my therapist often. In September of that same year, 2015, I was blessed to find a job for a local school district as a contract OT in a Minneapolis sub- urb. I was surrounded by a generous, kind, God-loving faculty that welcomed me with open arms, not knowing all that I had been though in the recent months and years. I felt that God was truly looking out for me, bringing this good fortune my way. To make matters even better, the school district had a high per- centage of people of color, and so for the first time, I felt truly at home working there. I was one of many, not an odd one out. You might wonder why an adult needed to feel like she fit in. To that I would say, no matter what your age, your experience, or your gender, it is a human reaction to want to fit in. And so, at fifty-three years old, the fact that I was surrounded by a more balanced number of people of color made me feel lighter than I ever had. Never underestimate the power of "fitting in." My principal made all the difference in affirming my skills and my heart for loving the children we worked with. The healing I gained from working in this district is priceless in my life and I will always be grateful. After reaching rock bottom, my life was on the upswing.

There's a quote that springs to mind here: "Sometimes you have to get knocked down lower than you ever have been to stand up taller than you ever were."

The quote is of unknown origins, for those of you wondering, but that doesn't make it any less perfect! And if this quote doesn't summarize my life perfectly, then nothing else ever will.

Excitingly, my youngest daughter graduated from high school a year later in June 2016. We'd gone through so much together, as she was the one riding the waves with me. We both had to learn what it meant to live in a one-parent household, with a mom who was suffering from mental illness. For me, her graduation signified that no matter my flaws, my kids turned out okay. Better than okay, and that is truly a blessing. After all we'd weathered together, in a turbulent time, we both became strong women together. Often, in times when I'm feeling that worthlessness trying to rear its ugly head, I look at my children and know that I've achieved great things with my life. As life continued onward, I felt the different strands begin to pull together. As I stand back and observe it all, I see how the strands are forming my ultimate hat woven together with all my experiences. Things started looking up for me. I learned about my condition and took the necessary steps to prevent myself from falling like I had before. I focused on how proud I was that I was able to get back on my feet after such a huge setback.

Confucius once said, "Our greatest glory is not in never falling, but in rising every time we fall." You can't argue with that logic! As my children all went in their own directions, I decided to do what I could to get on top of my seasonal affective disorder—go toward the sun. In July 2016, I sold almost all of my belongings, which made feel lighter and freer and ready for an adventure. I packed up my SUV with only what I could fit in the trunk and moved to South Florida for a professor position at a college. I started over, a brand-new chapter of my life. I remember walking on a beach once I arrived near the apartment I had rented and watching the waves come toward me and then flow back to the large ocean. I felt my troubles float away from the large sea of difficulties I had just left, finally turning the page on all the suffering and allowing myself to accept all the good that would come. This is a poem that I wrote at the time I moved to the sun-drenched shores of Florida, ready to start my new chapter. Two short lines for key catalysts in my life...

I know this to be true...

6/1980
I know this to be true:
I AM smart and I WILL be somebody.

2/1990
I know this to be true:
This baby will be the greatest creation I will ever be a part of.

6/1992
I know this to be true:
A baby girl to teach pride of her body and mind.

5/1994
I know this to be true:
Words can hurt and wound.

4/1996
I know this to be true:
I am not done and I will have another baby.

5/1996
I know this to be true:
Passion may come, in time, with this friend.

2/1998
I know this to be true:
I am blessed to be a mommy again.

3/2000
I know this to be true:
I have done my best, now I am numb.

6/2008
I know this to be true:
He is leaving soon but will return again.

9/2010
I know this to be true:
She WILL be okay.

12/2010
I know this to be true:
My child will be whole again.

7/2012
I know this to be true:
Your heart is made up of tiny pieces of your child's emotions.

9/2012
I know this to be true:
I will deeply love before I die.

12/2012
I know this to be true:
God is THE love of my life.

3/2013
I know this to be true:
Today is not the last day of my life. He loves me as HIS daughter and He is in control.

5/2013
I know this to be true:
I am not broken and I am worthy.

1/2014
I know this to be true:
"I am imperfect and I am enough."

4/2014
I know this to be true:
This marriage will be different; this marriage will be His gift to us.

6/2014
I know this to be true:
He was not THE one for me. After the pain has healed, I will be whole again.

9/2014

I know this to be true:

HE is my savior, my protector, and my constant, when all else fails.

6/2016

I know this to be true:

She is amazing and kind and wonderful and graduating.

8/2016

I know this to be true:

My baby has grown up and she will be just fine on her own and so will I.

10/2016

I know this to be true:

Chapter Two has so many hopes and dreams to come true.

What do you know to be true?

_____

_____

_____

_____

_____

_____

_____

_____

_____

_____

_____

_____

I have to admit that the progression through my life is something I am proud of. That even when I was at the lowest points, I got back up, dusted myself off, and carried on. It was never easy, but it was required to live again. This is something every single one of us does in our lives. We all face different things, different trials and tribulations, and we come out on the other side. You may face a different journey than I have, but we understand how hard those journeys can be. Our suffering is not relative. If you get up from your lowest times, celebrate that. No matter what your low is, you get up and get on with it (maybe after a good cry, scream, or tantrum).

✖ ✖ ✖ ✖ ✖

THE OTHER SIDE

learned to make the most of my time in South Florida. I began to get some semblance of myself again. I knew I was strong on my own. I started to figure out what hats I wanted to wear now, figuratively speaking of course. With Florida heat, hats are a welcome addition. You see, for the most part, my children didn't need me anymore. We were still close, but they didn't need my mothering anymore. They were adults after all. And so, I had to figure out who I was, not as a mother, or a wife, or even as a professional. Who was I? I lived just blocks from the beach, and I started to date and make friends; life was becoming comfortable. That's not to say I didn't have to take steps to take care of myself; mental health will always be a part of my life, but it was no longer at the forefront. I could make decisions without wondering whether my illness had caused me to react in a certain way. I made the most of being a single, care-free woman living in a beautiful area with great friends and a stable job. I was lucky and I knew it! The ocean helped to heal all the hurts of the past. I would have never suspected that the ocean could have the power to do that. But it did. My worries, embarrassments, and sadness went out with the tide, washing away the things that could no longer hurt me.

December 2016 was when things changed again. For the better this time, don't worry! My story is far from a fairy tale, but if you are a fan of happy endings, my story may please you. The day after Christmas, I received an unexpected phone call. My cell phone buzzed as I was just getting ready to leave a store parking lot. I didn't recognize the number and so I let it go to voicemail. Expecting a telemarketer or a sales call on the other end, I was pleasantly surprised to hear a voice from my past. As I listened to the message, a smile began to spread across my face. Alone, in my car, I couldn't stop grinning. The message was from my old high school boyfriend, the older boy my mother hated me dating, the one she was sure would make me pregnant. Remember him? Well, my mom has long since made any of my decisions, so I had no excuses. I recognized his voice instantly, a voice I hadn't heard since high school. I often wondered what had happened to him. Where was that high school boy that cared for my heart so many years ago? Did he have a happy life? Did he remain in Arizona after going to college there? Did he find joy in this journey called life? I never knew, but I was living my life to my fullest and hoped that he was doing the same. I always wished the best for him. Always. As it transpired, I knew I would have to move south after my youngest graduated from high school to help with my seasonal affective disorder, so I visited four different southern states and Arizona was one of those states. While in Phoenix, Arizona, I decide to take a chance and I sent an email to him, hoping to meet his wife and his children and really just to catch up with an old friend. Time passed, but there was no response. In December of 2016, he finally opened that email, which he had not checked in years. After my sweet email sat untouched, unviewed, in his spam collecting dust for years, he just did not recognize my married name from my email account. He describes the gnawing feeling of finally having to open that annoying email that had been there for years, yet never deleted it for some reason. He scrolled through the entire email to the very bottom of the letter only to finally see my maiden name and phone number under the email signature. He's always described that moment as losing his ability to breathe for a second. He had no choice, he reports, but to give that high school girl a phone call the day after Christmas.

I was so nervous to return the phone call. I felt like my stomach was full of butterflies trying to escape out of my skin. I felt exactly the same as I had the first time he called me and I answered on my princess phone, all those years ago. I needed courage. I was a grown woman, but I regressed to being that shy sophomore girl again. I quickly reached out to my sister, who had sat with me on my childhood bed as I cried after we had broken up. "You will never guess who I just got a voice-mail from?" "Who?" she asked. "Just tell me," she begged. "Who do I consider as 'the one who got away'?" I asked. "DAN? Are you kidding me?" she screamed in the phone blaring in my ear.

Just the reaction I had hoped. She knew me better than anyone. "What are you doing calling me? CALL HIM!! Hurry up, then call me back. Do it!" she screamed and giggled. With my heart in my throat, I called him back. I admit that I felt a pang of excitement when he told me he'd never married. The excitement turned to a little bit of jealousy (I'm only human!) when he told me he was in a relationship, but it was rocky. I'm terrible, but my smiled returned. We talked for over an hour. Promising to keep in touch, we eventually hung up the phone. I'd told him that I visited Arizona yearly, and we would meet up the next time I was in town. I too was in a relationship at the time, but it too was not going well. Dan and I both knew nothing could come of our reconnection, but it was so refreshing to speak to such a kind voice from my past. After a number of hurricanes hit South Florida, a job change, and a hard break-up with my then boyfriend, I decided that it was time to move again, as I was free to do. It was July 2017 when I took the plunge and packed up my car again, moving to Arizona to work as an OT with babies. Of course, I hoped to start dating my high school boyfriend again when I moved, but it was in God's hands at this point. He too had recently gone through a break-up and it seemed like the stars were aligning for us.

"Dare to live the life you have dreamed for yourself.
Go forward and make your dreams come true."

—Ralph Waldo Emerson

**Have you ever considered your own wildest dreams?
What are they, and how would they change your life?**

_____

_____

_____

_____

_____

_____

_____

You'll be pleased to know that I found hope again and found love as well. It all had to begin with me loving me again. I had to know I was strong on my own. Healing takes time, but it is possible.

It's been over three years now sharing my life with my high school boyfriend (as I still call him). He is still funny, loving, and charming, and makes me feel worthy. He is everything I ever dreamed of having with another person; it just took us a little bit longer than we would have liked to find each other again. Are things easy? Of course not. At our age we not only have baggage, we also have the carry-on and the large trunks along for the journey. But it works. I now live in a state where I look like so many others. I don't feel quite so different. Do I still hear racist remarks? Sure! But in a state where people of color are in the majority, rather than the minority, it doesn't sting quite like it used to. It took a lot of healing for me to realize that it is their problem not mine. I still don't like mean people, but I am stronger than I've ever been. I'm a professor and program director at a college now, and I run a private practice for children, adolescents, and young adults going through mental health difficulties in life. I like where I am in life. I like my job, my family, my partner. Has life been easy? No! Has it been an adventure? Absolutely! Would I ever change the color of my skin, my battles with depression, eating disorders, and body issues? Or the trials I have been through or the beautiful journey to get me to where I am today? No way. I'm blessed beyond measure to be living on the other side.

✕ ✕ ✕ ✕ ✕

THE LIGHT AT THE END
OF THE TUNNEL

So, that's me. That's my story. I am the sum of all my parts. Everything I told you has led me to where I am today. When the road seems rocky, or even unpassable, I want you to think of my story, how I've been down many rocky roads and yet find paved, smooth spots in my path so much more. I now find joy in small things. I give myself grace and attempt to choose happiness whenever I can. I hope that you find your happiness sooner than I did, but there's no limit on when you can change your life for the better. Whether you're seventeen or seventy, you can change your life. You too can put the wheels in motion to be happy. For some that might be reaching out to family that you haven't spoken to in years, getting rid of an awful boyfriend, or maybe even quitting a joy-sucking job. Our paths are different, it's what makes being human so exciting. It's also what makes being human so difficult. Please hold on and don't give up. You are stronger than you may know and you CAN do this.

"It is never too late to be what you might have been."

—**George Eliot**

And for the late bloomers out there, like me:

"There is nothing better in life than being a late bloomer.
Success can happen at any time and at any age. You can
have a spiritual awakening and discover a new side of
yourself. And best of all, love can happen at any age."

—**Salma Hayek**

How's that for inspirational?! #inspired, right?

The next section will be addressing self-help and strategies I have used with clients and things I wish I had told myself to use. At times, it seems easier to care for others than it is to care for yourself. You may have all the skills, all the tools, and all the advice, the counsel to give to others, but to take your own advice and use those skills on yourself, we seem to lose our way, we lose our confidence and just don't do it. I share with you things I wish I'd done, advice I wish I would have laid on my own ears, here for you to consider adding into your own lives. Knowledge is power, my friends. And with power comes the ability to change your life for the better. Don't worry, it's not going to be a prescriptive "you must do this, this, and this" in order to get better. I cannot tell you what to do. I can only let you know what may help. I can only let you know I care; I get it. What I'm going to share with you are things that I have done that might work for you. They also might not. You have my permission now to grasp hold of what works for you and throw away what doesn't. I won't be offended. I'm a strong woman, remember! We're all different, and different things work for each of us. What I offer are simply things you can try that might help you understand your mental illness, get the courage to reach out for help, or simply make small changes to take care of your mental health. I'm coming to this with real-world experience, as a mother, a professional, and somebody who has been through the ringer.

Reflect upon my story. How has it made you feel? Have you learned anything?

_____

_____

_____

_____

_____

_____

_____

_____

_____

_____

_____

✖ ✖ ✖ ✖ ✖

A GUIDE TO SUPPORTING YOUR MENTAL HEALTH AND WELL-BEING

THE SELF-HELP PORTION OF THE MENU

"To be a good parent, you need to take care of yourself so that you can have the physical and emotional energy to take care of your family."

—Michele Obama

This section is not only for parents or people taking care of others but also for those caring for themselves. The advice and hopefully useful information I share with you can be applied to all people, no matter what their circumstances. However, there are a couple of paragraphs at the end of this chapter that are solely about parenting with a mental health condition, just because that is my own area of experience and the road I most recently journeyed through. The rest is generic, so whether you are single, coupled, have fur babies, have no children, or your house is full of little ones, you can still gain a lot from this self-help section of the book. This self-help section aims to give you the tools you need to find what works for you. Like a lunch buffet, take what appeals to you and leave the rest for the people behind you. Only you can decide what the right path is for your own mental wellness. What works for me might not work for you. And that's absolutely okay. By giving my suggestions a go, and running with them or dumping them, you're a step closer to finding what works for you.

"It is so important to take time for yourself and find clarity. The most important relationship is the one you have with yourself."

—Diane Von Furstenberg

✖ ✖ ✖ ✖ ✖

A BRIEF OVERVIEW OF THE WORLD OF MENTAL HEALTH

Mental Health And Mental Illness Are Different Things

"Be confused, it's where you begin to learn new things. Be broken,
it's where you begin to heal. Be frustrated, it's where you start to
make more authentic decisions. Be sad, because if we are brave
enough we can hear our heart's wisdom through it. Be whatever
you are right now. No more hiding. You are worthy, always."

—S.C. Lourie

The World Health Organization has stated that, "There is no health without mental health." So, what is mental health? Mental health is everything pertaining to our mental well-being. It's our emotions, our feelings and thoughts, our ability to problem solve and overcome difficult situations, our social connections, and our understanding of the world. Sounds like a lot, doesn't it? That's because it is. Mental health is the umbrella term for where we sit on the continuum of our mental well-being. It's a spectrum and we all sit somewhere along it. Our place on the spectrum is fluid and changes consistently. This reminds me of a quote I read.

"Mental health is not a destination, but a process. It's about how you drive, not where you are going."

—Noam Shpancer

On this spectrum, or journey, we have a myriad of information, and that's okay. It's how we learn to cope with the place we land on the spectrum.

So, mental illness is different from mental health. It comes under the umbrella of mental health, but it is something entirely separate. A mental illness is a diagnosed illness. Just the same as having disease attacking your body, a mental illness wages war on our mind. Mental illness impacts the way a person thinks, feels, and behaves, and how they interact with others. There are a great many mental illness diagnoses that may have different impacts upon people. These diagnoses can be manageable and treatable and you should 100 percent, without a shadow of a doubt, seek medical attention just as you would if you broke your leg!

"At the root of this dilemma is how we view mental health in this country. Whether an illness affects your heart, your leg or your brain, it's still an illness, and there should be no distinction."

—Michelle Obama

What does mental health mean to you?

_____

_____

_____

_____

_____

Of course, there are other things that prevent people from seeking medical help too, including the availability of treatment, the cost of treatment, the symptoms of their illness preventing them from seeking treatment, they don't think their condition is "bad enough" (this one breaks my heart), they are scared of the treatment, and the big one: the stigma, embarrassment, and shame. If there's only one thing you take from reading this book and sharing in my story, it is that there is _no shame_ in having a mental illness. There is no shame in seeking treatment. Repeat that with me, there is no shame in having a mental illness. There is no shame in seeking treatment. Seeking help may be just the start of learning to manage mental illness. Seeking help is the bravest thing you may ever do.

Read this beautiful quote by Nido Qubein, and you'll understand exactly what I mean: "Your present circumstances don't determine where you can go; they merely determine where you start."

I don't believe that there's anything I can say that will make you go out and seek help. I don't know your story. I don't know what you suffer from or your circumstances. But I do know this; you are worth it. You are worth the treatment and the effort to work on your mental well-being. Nobody is a lost cause. Nobody, I repeat. You are so worth it!

"You, yourself, as much as anybody in the entire universe, deserve your love and affection." The Buddha said that, and if the Buddha said it, then you can't argue! It's true.

While I would love to go into the specifics of each mental illness with you, it is simply not feasible in this book. I'm not sure it would be particularly useful either, as each of these illnesses can present differently in different people. What depression looks like in me might be worlds away from how it looks in you. So, what I would like to include here instead, if you'll bear with me a moment, are a few common signs of mental illness. That way you'll have the information you need to make informed choices about your own mental health. If you see the following signs and think, "Yes, that's me!" or "Yes, that's my loved one!" then the best thing you can do is to seek help. It is very rare that a mental illness will suddenly happen out of the blue, and instead the symptoms tend to build, like a snowball rolling down a hill, gathering more snow. You might start to feel "not quite right." This is such a common feeling in people whose mental health is perhaps declining. Learning what symptoms to watch out for can help you to jump into action and seek the help.

Common Signs of Mental Illness

➤ **Sleep or appetite changes.** This includes both sleeping too much and sleeping too little, and, of course, eating too much or eating too little. Anything that is different to the norm for you. Similarly, along with this, you might notice a decline in personal care.

➤ **Mood changes.** This isn't just necessarily feeling down and depressed. It could be rapid changes in mood, or dramatic changes in mood. It can be feeling emotions that don't feel quite appropriate for what is going on around you too.

➤ **Withdrawal.** Whether that be from social activities or any interests you have.

➤ **Drop in functioning.** Your work performance might dip, or your grades. Or maybe you're quitting out of clubs, etc.

➤ **Problems thinking.** This is pretty self-explanatory. Sometimes you might struggle to think clearly, or your memory becomes distorted. Potentially, your logical thought might also become impaired.

➤ **Increased sensitivity.** This covers all five of the senses: taste, touch, sight, smell, and sound. It can lead to avoiding situations where you find certain stimuli overwhelming.

→ **Apathy.** A loss of desire or initiative to participate in activities.

→ **Feeling disconnected.** This is often one of the hardest to deal with, in my own opinion. You might feel disconnected from both yourself or your surroundings. Some people also find it hard to know what is real and what isn't.

→ **Illogical thinking.** Thinking that does not make sense. It may be grandiose. It may be impulsive, but it is illogical. You may have exaggerated beliefs about your personal powers or influence.

→ **Nervousness.** This isn't simply being nervous about an event. It's more all-encompassing. You might have a general feeling of nervousness all the time. You might feel suspicious of people or events, more so than you usually would. It might even feel like dread.

→ **Unusual behavior.** This is anything that you might classify as odd or uncharacteristic for you.

I hear all you busy folks out there saying that you don't have time to form a relationship with yourself, practice self-care, and take your mental health seriously. Neither did I, and look where it got me. Before I started to take care of myself, I wound up in the very place I hoped I never would: a psychiatric unit. And let me tell you something, if you can take steps to avoid ending up behind those double doors, then you definitely should. Your mental health is not something to shrug off or something to take care of "when you have more time." I'm not, however, unrealistic. I do know that life gets in the way and before we know it we're in our sunset years thinking, "What the hell happened?" and "Where did all that grey hair come from?"

Taking care of yourself isn't a full-time job, it is a gift we get to participate in every day. We'll talk about ideas toward recovery in this chapter, but we'll also cover general maintenance. Think of your mental health like your car. You have to fill it with fuel, service it, get new wiper blades, and vacuum it—all the responsibilities that come with car ownership. But you don't have to do all these every single day. You might if you allow your car to go neglected for a long period. But if you keep up with general maintenance, it only takes a little time. This is true for caring for your mental health as well. If you care for yourself little by little, then an "engine overhaul" may be avoided. We'll cover both maintenance and recovery, so that we've covered all our bases. Expect some activities to make you reflect on your mental wellness and/or mental health journey. By telling you my whole story, I want you to feel comfortable beginning to wade into the waves of your own mental health. Believe me when I say that I know as well as anyone that reflecting on your mental health isn't always an easy feat, especially if we have trauma we'd rather not deal with. The brain is complex, and this can make it difficult to take charge of your own mental health, no matter how much you want to. But the more you flex your self-care muscles, the more you will get to know what makes your brain tick and what makes it stutter. Now, the necessary disclaimer (I know you already know, but…), nothing I say here is meant to replace mental health treatment. Whether those treatments be therapy, medications, or holistic approaches, you need to seek proper treatment if you are suffering from mental health concerns. I wish more than anything that I can make everybody understand the importance of proper medical care. I have no room for judgment nor negative feelings about seeking medical attention or seeing a licensed therapist. It is a necessary, and often lifesaving, avenue of treatment. Just do it!

As Stephen Fry says in his ever-knowing wisdom, "The uncomfortable, as well as the miraculous, fact about the human mind is how it varies from individual to individual. The process of treatment can therefore be long and complicated…"

I think that this often puts people off from seeking treatment too, as well as the stigmas attached to the illness; people know that the mind is complicated and therefore finding the right treatment for you is complicated. Lord knows I know this all too well. But that feeling you get when you find the right balance of treatments can be so freeing. I'm not saying get yourself on medication, but I'm not saying avoid medication. For many people it works incredibly well, and for others it doesn't. If you need it, you need it. If you don't, you don't. You do what works for you, but if you need to seek medical attention then get your butt out the door and do it. You can even do what I did. Tell your friends or family what to watch out for—maybe for you it would be something different from my red flags of talking about my children being better off without me—and when they notice your signs they can push you to get help. Of course, that might not be driving you to the nearest emergency room, it might be supporting you to make an appointment with your doctor or a therapist. Just know that when you feel yourself descending into something that seems out of your control, there should be no ifs or buts to get help. Period. Not to sound harsh, but I've seen poor outcomes more times than I would have liked. And, without my friends, I too would have been another statistic.

"Just because no one else can heal or do your inner work for you doesn't mean you can, should, or need to do it alone."

—Lisa Olivera

Yes, I've put this quote in bold because it's pretty important. Healing your mental health is never something you have to, or should do alone. But you need to put in the work too. It's not something anybody can fix for you, even if they have the best of intentions. It takes work to get better. Think of it like seeing an athletic trainer after taking a break from exercise; it will take a while (and a lot of hard work!) to get back into tip-top shape, and even then you might never get back to peak condition, but you'll be so much healthier than before. The same goes for your mental health. Just as an athletic trainer guides you through exercises to get your body working as well as it can, a mental health therapist will do the same with your mind. If you have the means to explore therapy, even when you are not struggling with your mental health, I would 100 percent recommend giving it a go.

Anyway, enough of my rambling about how important it is to seek help (I bet I sound like your mother!) let's get down to the nitty gritty of this chapter, the things you can do to take care of your mental well-being.

What do you do to take care of yourself?

_____

_____

_____

_____

_____

_____

"The idea that you have to be protected from any kind of uncomfortable emotion is what I absolutely do not subscribe to."

—John Cleese

✖ ✖ ✖ ✖ ✖

SELF-CARE THROUGH JOURNALING

I f you couldn't have guessed already, I'm a huge journaling nerd. Shock, horror! When people think of journaling, they often visualize that little girl with a pink diary and glitter gel pens with a tiny lock on the front cover, but that's not what we're talking about here. Your journal could be drawings or sketches of feelings. I use words, but the choice is yours. You don't have to start with "Dear Diary," or anything like that, unless you want to (who am I to judge?). Journaling has long since been proven to have clinical benefits for people with mental illnesses.[4] It is real. It is scientifically proven, and I can personally vouch that it works. I am a success story of journaling. I have used it with a great many patients, hundreds in fact.

---

4 Miller, William. "Interactive journaling as a clinical tool." *Journal of Mental Health Counseling* 36, no. 1 (2014): 31-42; Ullrich, P.M. and Lutgendorf, S.K., "Journaling about stressful events: Effects of cognitive processing and emotional expression," *Annals of Behavioral Medicine*, 24(3) (2002), pp.244-250; Smyth, J.M., Johnson, J.A., Auer, B.J., Lehman, E., Talamo, G. and Sciamanna, C.N., "Online positive affect journaling in the improvement of mental distress and well-being in general medical patients with elevated anxiety symptoms: a preliminary randomized controlled trial," *JMIR mental health*, 5(4) (2018), p.e11290.

There's no right or wrong way to journal. Whether you pick up pen and paper, buy a fancy notebook, or use your laptop, as long as your brain is processing the words you are writing, then you're certain to get some benefit from it. If you're a skeptic, and I don't blame you, I'd like you to give it a go (for me!) and see what happens. If you don't like it after you've tried it, then throw it in a dumpster and move onto something else. This section is a precursor to self-care and maintenance of your mental health, but it's so important that I wanted to give it the spotlight I think it deserves.

Journaling has been proven to have tons of benefits, too many for me to list here. But the main ones I'd like to share with you are:

➜ Boost in your mood.
➜ Enhanced sense of well-being.
➜ Reduced symptoms of depression before an important event.
➜ Reduced intrusion and avoidance symptoms of post-trauma.
➜ Improvement to working memory.
➜ A shift in negative mind-set.
➜ Improved self-awareness.[5]

Who wouldn't want these benefits?

While there are no concrete rules to journaling, there are some tips that you might want to follow to make it work for

5 Baikie, K.A. and Wilhelm, K., "Emotional and physical health benefits of expressive writing," *Advances in psychiatric treatment*, 11 (5) (2005), pp.338-346.

you. Again, you do you. You don't have to follow any of these tips if you don't feel like it.

1. Write in a private and comfortable space, free from distractions.
2. Aim to write at least once each day, consecutively if you can.
3. Allow yourself time to reflect before and after you write.
4. If you're writing to overcome trauma or bad experiences, you don't have to write about that specific event. Just journal what feels right to you.
5. Structure the writing whatever way feels right.
6. Keep the journal for your eyes only. This will stop you filtering your feelings and experience. I would suggest not even showing it to your therapist. You can share what you've written aloud, but keep the journal for you.

✖ ✖ ✖ ✖ ✖

THERE ARE TONS OF JOURNAL PROMPTS OUT THERE

I'll share some with you, but if you're not one for prompts then you could try the WRITE method for journaling. This can give you a bit of structure that can be helpful when you're starting out.

- **What** do you want to write about? Spent time thinking about what you want to write about.
- **Reflect** upon the topic you've chosen. Consider the who, what, when, where, why around the topic. Start writing.
- **Investigate** your thoughts about the topic. Continue writing. Try not to think too hard on your words, just let them pour out and onto the paper. If you get stuck, take a second, read what you've written, and carry on.

➜ **Time** yourself writing. Make sure the exercise lasts for at least five minutes each time. You can choose a time limit that works for you. It doesn't have to be five minutes.

➜ **Exit** in a strategic way. Don't just stop writing, ending your train of thought when the timer goes off. Make sure you finish with a reflective statement. Re-read what you've written again and write a little summary sentence or two to end it nicely.

Now that we've got that out of the way, let's get down to business. I love a good thought-provoking journal prompt! A quick Google search for 'Journal prompts for...' (you fill in the blank) will bring up loads of prompts you can explore. Try adding in "depression," "anxiety," "stress," or "recovery" to the end of the sentence for more specific journaling options. For me, I'm going to keep it generic here, outlining ones that can benefit everyone, I hope. They're some of my personal favorites!

- Write down as many things as you can that make you incredibly happy. Why does each one make you feel this way?

- Write a letter to a person that has positively impacted you (you don't have to send it).

- Write a poem about who you are. Write a poem about somebody who is the opposite of you.

- Write about one of your happiest memories.

- In detail, write about a perfect day (real or imagined).

- Write a list of all the things you'd like to remember during difficult times.

- Write a letter of forgiveness to yourself.

- Write a list of your regrets. Either throw them away, or throw them into the fire.

- Write a letter to future you.

- Write a letter to past you.

- Describe an outfit that makes you feel completely comfortable in your own skin.

- What are some of your favorite books? Write about them.

- Describe your dream house. Focus on all five senses.

- Write a love letter to yourself.

- Write about something that's holding you back. How are you going to overcome it?

- What speaks to you on a spiritual level? Why do you feel this way?

- Write a letter of forgiveness to somebody that has caused you pain.

- What do you wish others knew about you?

- What song helps to lift your mood when you're feeling down?

- Create a list of things you want to achieve in the next twelve months.

- What is the biggest lesson in life you've learned to date?

- What do you want your future to look like?

You can also use quotes or scripture as the basis for your journaling. This is something I love to do. It's nice to have a change of scenery once in a while, don't you think? Here are a few quotes you could use. A quick Google search for "quotes about…" will bring up a lot of options too if these don't speak to you.

"What in your life is calling you? When all the noise is silenced, the meetings adjourned, the lists laid aside, and the wild iris blooms by itself in the dark forest, what still pulls on your soul? In the silence between your heartbeats hides a summons, do you hear it? Name it, if you must, or leave it forever nameless, but why pretend it is not there?"

—The Terma Collective

"Most people are other people. Their thoughts are someone else's opinions, their lives a mimicry, their passions a quotation."

—Oscar Wilde

"To forgive is to set a prisoner free and discover that the prisoner was you."

—Lewis B. Smedes

Of course, the list could be endless. There are lots of prompts on the internet, and you can also buy guided journals that provide prompts for each day if you'd like a bit of structure. Just search for "guided journals" and you'll find a huge list. Some favorites are *The Five-Minute Journal*, *52 Lists for Happiness*, and *Q&A a Day: 5-Year Journal*, although there are tons to choose from.

If you don't mind, I'd like to share with you a day from my journal. The prompt was to write a letter to the past you. I like to answer the journal questions through poetry. I don't know why, but it just works for me. So this is what I wrote...

An Email to the Little Inside

———————

I wish I could email the Little that still resides inside of me.

*I'm all grown up on the outside, but deep inside in the corners
of my deep self lies the Little that dares not come out.*

*I would tell my Little how amazing and lucky she is. I would tell her that although
it seems scary and evil, the world can and does offer some pretty incredible things!*

*I know my Little longs to try adventures and take a risk, but no,
she would never because what would my friends think?*

*I know my Little would love to take a chance at love again, but no, the
scabs have barely healed from the last time that step was attempted.*

*I know my Little longs to step out of the box, to break the rules for once,
but no, she's a good girl and does exactly what is expected at all times.*

I also know my Little is slowly dying from not seeing the light of day.

*She needs to be let out. She needs exposure. She needs to be given a
chance to grow and flourish. She needs the courage to try.*

My email would say,

*"Please take a chance. Please step out before it is too late. Although
you have seen hurt and although you have seen pain, the world
has so much more to offer that you need to experience."*

I would go on to say,

"It's ok. I'm all grown up and I will be right there beside you.

I won't leave you to do this alone."

How you journal is entirely up to you, but I would certainly love for you to give it a go. As you can see, you can choose to answer the prompts in whatever way you like. Or go rogue and don't use prompts at all. Journaling can be a great way to get in touch with your feelings and work through any issues you are facing, so give it a go and see what happens.

Write an email to your younger self.

_____

_____

_____

_____

_____

_____

_____

_____

_____

_____

_____

✗ ✗ ✗ ✗ ✗

MAINTENANCE AND SELF-CARE

For a lot of people out there, mental health isn't necessarily about recovering from a mental illness, it's about maintaining and taking care of your mental health and well-being. Just because you've never suffered from a mental illness doesn't mean that self-care and maintaining your health isn't super important. You can also take care of your mind. Healthy eating and exercise are great ways to keep your mind healthy as well as your body. A double whammy! You're welcome. Maintaining good mental health often comes in the same boat as self-care. This is a pretty new phrase and is something that you'll hear a lot when you begin to delve into the world of mental health. Self-care is the means by which we can both improve our mental health (along with other appropriate treatments for any disorders) and maintain our mental health. Self-care is any activity that we do deliberately in order to take care of our mental, emotional, and physical health. It is not a selfish act; it is something that allows us to refuel in order to carry on. It's all about knowing what we need to do in order to take care of ourselves and therefore do all the other things we need to do in life. You can't pour from an empty cup. Thinking back to my story, for years I tried to pour from an empty cup, and it wasn't until I stopped and started to take care of myself that I realized self-care was what I needed to do in order to have something in my cup to pour.

There are three golden rules to self-care. Self-care is not at all a complicated task, but so often I have seen people make it so complicated, giving a list of rules we need to follow in order for something to be classed as self-care. And that's just not the case at all. There are three things you need to consider with self-care, and that's it. I will give you some ideas on what might be self-care, but at the end of the day it's all down to you and what fills your cup.

1. **Keep it simple.** Don't try too much too soon. Try to implement a couple of things into your existing routine that make you feel good. Then you can begin to increase self-care behaviors over time.

2. **You have to plan for it.** The point of self-care is that it is deliberate. Plan into your diary, tell others what you are doing to take care of yourself, whatever it takes to make your plan concrete. Whether you plan ten minutes into your day to read a book, or block out two hours each week for a bubble bath, it doesn't matter. Just get it planned and don't compromise.

3. **View what you are doing as necessary self-care.** Be conscious about it. Think about why you are doing it, how it makes you feel, and what the outcomes are.

✖ ✖ ✖ ✖ ✖

SOME THINGS YOU CAN INCLUDE IN YOUR SELF-CARE REGIMES ARE...

Healthy Eating and Exercise

I know that for loads of people, myself included, healthy eating and exercising can be a bit of a chore. I have to be careful that I don't fall into unhealthy thought patterns thanks to my eating disorder, but it doesn't have to be extreme. Something as simple as eating your five fruits and veggies each day and getting out of the house for a walk is often enough to keep your brain and your body ticking over nicely in that department. Exercise releases serotonin, which improves our mood, an added bonus for all of us I should think.

Make a "No List"

This could be a little activity for your journal. Your "no list" should include all of the things that you don't want to do, that make you feel miserable. You still have to go about your daily duties, of course, or our lives would simply stop. But things that you don't have to do, that you hate to do, stop doing them. You don't have to explain to anybody why you no longer answer work emails after 6 p.m. or why you don't attend gatherings with your judgmental mother-in-law. If it makes you unhappy and you don't have to do it, then don't. Get that list written and try to stick to it.

Get Enough Sleep

Sleep is something we often see as a luxury, especially those of us who are parents or carers. Sleep is not something that we can live without. Adults need at least seven to eight hours of sleep each night on average. Don't cheat yourself out of a good night's sleep. With a decent rest often we think more clearly and have an improved mood.

Your Planned Self-Care Activities

As a good rule of thumb, you should do one activity each day that relaxes you and one that you enjoy, so essentially two self-care activities. That's all. They don't have to last long, but you should try to plan for them. Having a good stretch or taking a walk for some might be a good relaxing activity. Similarly, activities that you enjoy (which make you happy) might be something like going to the movies or watching TV. We're all different and our cups are filled by different things.

Take Care of Medical Needs

Yes, this seems self-explanatory. But for people with mental illness, getting yourself to the doctors and follow-up appointments can be like running a marathon. Taking care of your medical needs is part of your self-care and is important to both maintain good mental health or recover from mental illness, no matter which category you fall into. It's not unusual to put off seeing the doctor, or other medical appointments, but it can be a huge boost to your well-being when you take charge!

Spend Time with Loved Ones

Notice I didn't say spend time with your family? For a lot of people their loved ones are entirely separate from their families; we shouldn't assume that people want to be around them. So, spend time with the people you love, whether they are friends or family, it doesn't matter. On that note, if you have a family member or friend that is somebody you don't want to be around for whatever reason, you can certainly do the opposite and stop spending time with them. You are not obliged to spend time with anybody you do not wish to.

✖ ✖ ✖ ✖ ✖

THE ONE-OFFS
(COMPLETED WITH A
GUILT-FREE ATTITUDE)

These are everyday self-care things you might choose to do—the fundamentals of self-care, if you will. But what about the one-off, or semi-regular self-care activities? The ones we plan into our diaries in advance to refill our cups? Well, there's loads of options there too. Check out some of these, and if they tickle your fancy, get them jotted down in your diary!

- Take a nap without an alarm.
- Learn a new skill.
- Rearrange or redecorate your living space.
- Read a novel.
- Try a new hobby.
- Join an exercise class.
- Buy an adult coloring book.
- Read a magazine.

➜ Listen to a podcast.

➜ Declutter something.

➜ Unplug from social media.

➜ Make a Spotify playlist for your current mood.

➜ Watch a sad film and cry.

➜ Try some mindfulness exercises (there are loads online).

➜ Write and recite some positive affirmations.

➜ Look at the stars.

➜ Listen to music.

➜ Spend time with animals.

➜ Make some art.

➜ Take yourself out for a meal.

➜ Go on a bike ride.

➜ Join a support group.

➜ Join a book club.

➜ Try your hand at some art or music therapy (as an OT this is something I love!)

Do you see that this list is endless too? If you have a moment, maybe make a list of all the self-care activities you'd like to try out. You might already have some go-to things that make you feel better, but give some new ones a try too. You'll likely surprise yourself!

What self-care one-offs are you going to try?

_____

_____

_____

_____

_____

_____

_____

_____

✕ ✕ ✕ ✕ ✕

MENTAL HEALTH AND YOUR FAMILY

We spoke about some statistics at the beginning of the book, and before we get into this section, I just want to reiterate some. When we start talking about being a parent with a mental illness, or parenting a child that has a mental illness, this can bring up some pretty intense feelings for many of us. Millions of Americans live with a mental illness, and forty-six million people have mental health conditions. That's a whopping one in five adults. You are not alone if you have a mental illness, not by any means. For me, because of my inclination toward mental illness, I put everything I had into parenting my children.

Parenting, or taking care of another person who is dependent on you, is a difficult job by any standards. I don't think there's a single person on the planet who would argue that parenting is easy, and if there is I would love to learn their secret. Often, if you find yourself struggling with mental health issues, no matter what they are, you'll find that parenting becomes a little bit harder (or a lot harder), just the same as if you were to parent with a chronic physical illness. This doesn't mean that you can't have a happy and healthy family. My children are incredible, and I had my own issues to contend with too. If I can do it, so can you! Whether you have a mental illness that severely impacts your daily life, or you have something that you currently manage well, here are some tips that I have found to be really useful for parenting with a mental illness:

1. **Start with recognizing your strengths as a parent.** All too often we get bogged down with what we do badly that we forget to celebrate what we do well. Of course you're going to fail in some aspects; what parent doesn't? But why focus on that when you're doing so many other things well. Not only does this help you to keep going, but it is a positive model for your children too. They see a lot more than we give them credit for and seeing a parent focusing on the positives and building upon them teaches them what it means to be resilient. Troubleshooting when things go wrong can also help you to move forward. Reflecting on your days, or at the very least what went well and what didn't, can help you to create a plan of action for the next day.

2. **You need to take care of yourself too.** All the items we talked about in terms of self-care are nonnegotiable. You're no use to anyone if you're not taking care of yourself. It's not selfish, it's not a waste of time. It's as

important as any of those other jobs you have to fit into your day. Similarly, you need to take care of your health needs. Whether that be seeking treatment for mental or physical symptoms, problems occur when you put off the inevitable. Engaging in treatment for your mental illness is the best way to ensure that your children and your family thrive. I can't emphasize that enough.

3. **Connect. Connect. Connect.** Join support groups, either real or online. Surrounding yourself with people who understand what you are going through can help you to feel a lot less isolated, and we all know that having a mental illness can feel really isolating at times. Having somebody to rant to, to laugh with, and to make you push forward when you're having a bad day is worth the world to parents. Even something as simple as joining a play group and befriending other parents (even those without mental illnesses, or those who don't admit to it) can help you to feel connected.

4. **Planning is key.** Only you know the extent of your mental illness, and I'm sorry for being a negative Nelly here, but this is important. You need to have a crisis plan in place should you have an emergency. It's good practice anyway as a parent to have a crisis plan in place but more so for parents with a mental illness. If you experience an exacerbation and have to be hospitalized, who will take care of your children? Even the act of planning this can take pressure off your shoulders. Even if you

think you'll never need to use it, it's nice to have that comfort blanket.

5. **Make the most of your time together.** That doesn't mean spending every single waking moment at the beck and call of your children; that's not what you should be aiming for. What I mean is through knowing yourself and your mental illness, you'll be aware of when you are likely to be at your best. Maybe it's in the evenings, weekends, or at 3:47 p.m. on a Wednesday, it doesn't matter. This is the time you should be planning for with your children. If you know that you get anxious traveling, then plan more things around the home. If you know that you get anxious in the evenings, then plan your self care around this time and allow your children some free time. A little free time is not going to hurt your children; in fact, it's very healthy! On a similar note, after-school activities can be a Godsend if you need more time to yourself to keep things under control.

We often skip over the positives of being a parent with a mental illness. Before you send the villagers after me with pitchforks screaming, "Mental illness isn't a good thing, Sandi!" I know that. I know that mental illness is scary, it's dark, it's unsettling, and it's awful most of the time, if truth be told. But something we never talk about is the compassion and resilience that parents with a mental illness have. I would suggest straight off the bat that you share with your child about your mental illness. Only you know how much detail to share with them and whether they're ready to understand it. Don't go into any of the gory details, of course. Your children are still kids! But maybe share with them that sometimes Mommy or Daddy's brain feels a little tired and so they need to rest, or sometimes Mommy feels a little scared of things she knows won't hurt her. You get my drift. When your mental illness gets the better of you (which it will, we're all human!) explaining to your children what happened and that you're sorry can go a long way. For example, say you lose your temper and shout about something (we've all done this, so no judgment, mental illness or not), simply saying, "Mommy/Daddy is sorry for shouting. I was frustrated/sad/confused (or anything else), it's not your fault and I'll try not to let it happen again," can go a long way. This shows that you are holding yourself accountable and not making excuses for your behaviors. It's okay to make mistakes.

Now, a quick talk about the compassion parents with mental illness have and how this can rub off on their children, I saw this on my own. With a mental illness you often see the world through a different light, like a strange superpower. You know what happens when the straw breaks the camel's back, and when you see people being angry, nasty, sad, you have the ability to see it as more than just another person's messed-up personality. You know that something is going on that has made them behave in a certain way. You model compassion to your children by the way you treat others and the way in which you treat yourself. Remember that children are little sponges and they see all the good you do even if you don't see it yourself. They also see it when you value yourself and your family, enough to ask for help. They don't see it as a sign of weakness; they see it as a useful tool, which it certainly is if we're being honest!

Whether you're a parent or not, has this changed your perspective on parenting with a mental illness?

_____

_____

_____

_____

_____

_____

_____

_____

_____

_____

✖ ✖ ✖ ✖ ✖

YOU'VE GOT THIS!

How can I be certain that you can go forth and handle anything life throws at you? Because you cared enough to read this book. You cared enough to listen to my story and my humble words of wisdom. When I say, "You've got this!" that isn't me being toxically positive, it's me being real. By taking ownership of your mental health (whether you have a mental illness or not) you put the power in your own hands. Only you can go and get great treatment, only you can practice self-care, only you can be kind and forgiving to yourself. If you need medicine to get better, go for it. If you need therapy, go for it. If you need to practice being kind and compassionate to yourself, you guessed it, go for it! Maybe a combination would work for you. Don't sit on the symptoms of a mental illness until they become unbearable. Hopefully this chapter has given you some insight into what you can do to take care of yourself, and therefore those around you, while also keeping your mind healthy. I know that you can do this because I did it. I'm a real-life example of reaching rock bottom and clawing my way back to the surface. I'm happier now than I have been in years, and I wish that for you too. It's not unattainable. It's not wishful thinking. George Lucas once said, "You simply put one foot in front of the other and keep going."

Reflect upon this chapter. What have you learned?

_____

_____

_____

_____

_____

_____

_____

_____

_____

_____

_____

_____

_____

_____

_____

_____

_____

✖ ✖ ✖ ✖ ✖

SUMMARY

COURAGE DOESN'T ALWAYS ROAR

"Courage doesn't always roar. Sometimes courage is the little voice at the end of the day that says I'll try again tomorrow."

—Mary Anne Radmacher

I saved the best quote for last, didn't I? Something about these words by Mary Anne Radmacher just speaks to my soul. The fact that courage isn't always some big act with fanfare and balloons, sometimes it's just as simple as waking up the next day and quietly doing our best, no matter what our best is. We're so lucky to be able to say, "I'll try again tomorrow." There was a brief time in my life when I almost gave up the chance to be able to say these words every day. Of course, I have bad days, we all have bad days, it's the nature of the game. But the courage to just keep on keeping on is what, I believe, makes the bravest people. I've shared my soul with you, my story, my poetry, and my words of advice, my counsel, and in doing so I feel that I am on this journey with you.

In the USA, over 50 percent of people will experience a mental illness at some point in their lives. There's a one in two chance that will be you. I'm not saying that to scare you; mental illness is not something to be scared of, because if treated you can keep it under control. I'm trying to be realistic here. The stigma around mental health, especially given that so many adults in the USA currently have mental illness, is absolutely unacceptable! It has been estimated that approximately 68 percent of women and 57 percent of men who suffer from a mental illness are parents. You know this. I mentioned this right at the start of the book, though I'm sure that feels like forever ago! The thing is, until we start normalizing living with mental illness, it's never going to get better. I know that's easy for me to say now that I've come out of the other side, but it's better late than never. Coming from the perspective of being a professional working with mental health, to being a parent while simultaneously having a mental illness to being admitted to a psychiatric unit, I think it's safe to say that my story is unique in many ways. But just like you, I'm somebody trying to figure out how to be happy and how to make the people that I love happy. That's all. Nothing more, nothing less.

Sometimes I think that I'm still that little brown girl trying to find my place in a world I don't yet understand. I believe everybody feels that way at some point or another. While you might not have faced the same demons as me, I'm sure you've faced your fair share too. I want my book to empower you to know that whatever life throws at you, you can get through it. It might be an absolute pain and just suck at times, but you can do it and you can live a life you want to live. You can be the person you want to be if you take ownership of your mental well-being and keep putting one foot in front of the other and get to the other side.

What are your next steps?

_____

_____

_____

_____

_____

_____

_____

_____

_____

_____

_____

_____

_____

_____

✗ ✗ ✗ ✗ ✗

RESOURCES

You are not alone. If you or someone you know needs help, please reach out. No Stigma, only Hope.

National Suicide Prevention Hotline (available 24 hours a day)
800-237-TALK (8255)

NAMI-National Alliance on Mental Illness
800-950-NAMI (6264)

TWLOHA-To Write Love on Her Arms
text TWLOHA to 741741

Veteran's Crisis Line
800-237-8255, press 1

Trevor Project Lifeline
800-488-7386

CPSIA information can be obtained
at www.ICGtesting.com
Printed in the USA
BVHW090956240521
608000BV00012B/3020